Obesity and Overweight Matters in Primary Care

D0551744

Ruth Chambers
and
Gill Wakley

With contributions from
Ian Campbell
David Haslam
and
Peter Stott

Foreword by
Ian Banks

Staffordshire
UNIVERSITY

RADCLIFFE MEDICAL PRESS

Radcliffe Medical Press Ltd
18 Marcham Road
Abingdon
Oxon OX14 1AA
United Kingdom

www.radcliffe-oxford.com
The Radcliffe Medical Press electronic catalogue and online ordering facility.
Direct sales to anywhere in the world.

British Library Cataloguing in Publication Data

A catalogue record for this book is available from the British Library.

ISBN 1 85775 514 6

616.398 CHA.

Typeset by Joshua Associates Ltd, Oxford
Printed and bound by TJ International Ltd, Padstow, Cornwall

Contents

Foreword

Ruth Chambers and Gill Wakley have long track records for high-lighting important issues in general practice. In this book they team up with experts in obesity, producing a book which, I suspect, will develop well-thumbed pages in a short space of time.

A quick scan through the chapter on the 'scale of the problem' gives some idea of the impact obesity is having on health, workload and finance. The rising level of childhood obesity is not just a medical time bomb, it is a national disgrace. Schools have been forced to sell off playing fields and cut their physical education programmes under pressure from the National Curriculum, whilst building car parks for parents running their children to school rather than allowing them to cycle on our lethal roads. Food advertising targeting young children has a lot to answer for. Such a sad irony, with more TV chefs than you can shake a ladle at extolling the virtues of 'healthy eating'. Yet for many lower income group parents, simply travelling to out-of-town shopping centres is financially punitive compared to using readily available fast food outlets.

At a time when workload and the lack of community health professionals are the two critical factors for the survival of general practice, nothing could be more apposite than the management of obesity. There is no shortage of 'moan and groan' publications but what we desperately need is a reliable, evidence-based workshop manual for managing obesity. This book fits the bill. As one of its eminent contributors, Ian Campbell, once said, 'I would rather treat a patient's obesity for a year than diabetes for the rest of their life'. Wise words indeed but made all the more poignant when the WHO declares that obesity is the greatest single threat to life expectancy in the developed world.

Patients may become statistics but numbers alone will never convey the preventable tragedy of obesity or the importance of medical intervention in the all-important setting of general practice.

Improving a person's life, protecting them from obesity-related conditions while making them feel better about themselves is no mean feat. When it comes to their body mass index (BMI), we want to see less of our patients, not more of them!

Ian Banks
President, Men's Health Forum
Chairman, European Men's Health Forum
September 2001

About the authors

Ruth Chambers has been a GP for 20 years and is currently the Professor of Primary Care Development at Staffordshire University. She has designed and organised many types of educational initiatives, including distance-learning programmes. She has developed a keen interest in working with GPs, nurses and others in primary care around clinical governance and continuing professional development plans. She is the Royal College of General Practitioners' Convenor of Accredited Professional Development and the NHS Alliance's education lead.

Ruth is co-authoring this new series of books designed to help readers to draw up their own personal development plans or practice learning plans focusing on important health-related topics, such as obesity. She has been interested in obesity throughout her career, since undertaking original research into adipose-cell size in relation to age of onset of obesity for her first degree.

Gill Wakley started in general practice in 1966, but transferred to community medicine shortly afterwards and then into public health. A desire for increased contact with patients caused a move back into general practice, together with community gynaecology, in 1978. She has been combining the two, in varying amounts, ever since. Throughout she has been heavily involved in learning and teaching. She was in a training general practice, became an instructing doctor and a regional assessor in family planning, and was until recently a Senior Clinical Lecturer with the Primary Care Department at Keele University. Like Ruth, she has run all types of educational initiatives and activities, from individual mentoring and instruction to small group work, plenary lectures, distance-learning programmes, workshops, and courses for a wide range of health professionals and lay people.

Ian Campbell is a general practitioner in Nottingham and a graduate of Glasgow University. He is Chair of the National Obesity Forum and clinical governance lead for Gedling PCG. His published work has centred around the need for obesity management in primary care. He has helped to develop an educational programme for obesity management in primary care, which is available through the National Obesity

Forum. He sits on several industry and editorial boards, and has advised health authorities on developing local obesity management strategies.

David Haslam is a general practitioner in rural Hertfordshire who qualified from St Thomas's Medical School in 1986. He has a special interest in obesity, including the history of corpulence and its treatment, and the attitude of society towards it over the years. He has published fairly widely on the topic. He is the vice-chair of the National Obesity Forum and author of their guidelines (*see* Appendix 2). He is currently involved in the formulation of guidelines for the management of childhood obesity.

Peter Stott has been a general practitioner in Tadworth, Surrey, for 25 years and is a member of the National Obesity Forum. He was previously a Research Fellow/Lecturer at Surrey University. He has long had an interest in lifestyle as it applies to health, particularly in relation to the management of obesity, a subject on which he has lectured extensively to both professional and lay audiences. He has been involved in clinical trials on obesity, and his practice currently runs a nurse-led obesity clinic.

Abbreviations

BMI   body mass index
CHD   coronary heart disease
CVD   cardiovascular disease
HA   health authority
HDL   high-density lipoprotein (cholesterol)
Hg   mercury
HImP   health improvement programme
IT   information technology
kcal   kilocalorie (1000 kcal are equivalent to 4.2 MJ)
LA   local authority
LDL   low-density lipoprotein (cholesterol)
MI   myocardial infarction
NHS   National Health Service
NNT   number needed to treat
PCG   primary care group
PCO   primary care organisation*
PCT   primary care trust
PDP   personal development plan
PPDP   practice personal and professional development plan
SWOT   strengths, weaknesses, opportunities and threats

* The term 'primary care organisation' includes primary care groups or trusts in England, local health groups in Wales, local healthcare co-operatives in Scotland, and local health and social care groups in Northern Ireland.

Introduction

Focus your continuing professional development on obesity and overweight

This book sets out how learning more about obesity and overweight and reviewing your current practice can be incorporated into your personal development plan or the practice learning plan.[1,2] You should make learning more about obesity a priority, as this condition is the cause of a great deal of preventable ill health and premature mortality. Obesity is so common in developed countries that it is now being described as reaching 'epidemic' proportions.

Box 1

'Obesity is a condition in which weight gain has reached the point of seriously endangering health. While some people are genetically more susceptible than others, the direct cause of obesity in any individual is always an excess of energy intake over energy expenditure.'[3]

You need to develop a dual focus on improving your management of obesity and improving the efficiency of your working environment in the practice. Primary care team members should work together to direct their individual personal learning plans to form their practice personal and professional development plan. This should complement the clinical governance and business plans of the practice or primary care organisation.[2]

Box 2 Key facts about obesity in England[3]

- About one in five adults is obese (21% of women and 17% of men).
- The incidence of obesity has trebled in the last 20 years.

- Obesity is estimated to account for 18 million days of sickness absence a year and 30 000 deaths a year, resulting in 40 000 lost years of working life.
- Deaths linked to obesity shorten life by 9 years on average.
- The estimated financial cost of obesity is a £0.5 billion a year in treatment costs to the NHS.

The challenges for general practice teams are as follows:

- to help to prevent children and adults from becoming overweight and then obese
- to help those who are already overweight or obese to lose weight and sustain that weight loss.

The magnitude of the task means that resources should be prioritised – that is, invested in effective interventions. In the past GPs have been reimbursed for measuring patients' weight and height as part of a 'well-person' check. However, this has been shown to be a pointless exercise, as almost all obese people who attend general practice already know that they are overweight – or could easily deduce that from their own information. Most of them also know that obesity carries health risks.[4]

You may decide to allocate 50% of the time you intend to spend drawing up and applying a personal development plan this year on learning more about obesity. That would leave space in your learning plan for other important topics such as mental health, diabetes or cancer – whatever is a priority for you, your post and your patient population. There will be some overlap between topics. For example, you cannot consider a person who is obese in isolation from their risk factors for diabetes, or cardiovascular disease or any established disease.

The first chapter of the book describes the scale of the problem in the UK population. The incorporation of a clinical governance culture into the effective management of individuals who are overweight or obese, supported by well-organised general practice systems, is covered in Chapter 2. You should be able to demonstrate that you are fit to practise as an individual clinician or manager (best practice in the management of obesity, in this case), and that your working environment is fit to practise from. This section will be relevant to all readers, whether you are a clinician or a primary care manager, so that you understand more of the context within which you work and how your individual contribution fits into the whole picture of healthcare.

Thereafter each chapter gradually builds up your knowledge base so that you can access the most recent evidence for prevention or effective interventions with regard to overweight and obesity. We usually cite evidence from a review or compendium rather than the original literature, for the sake of simplicity.

The whole programme builds up to the generation of a personal development plan and a practice personal and professional development plan in Chapters 10 and 11.[1] Interactive reflection exercises at the end of each chapter give the reader an opportunity to assess their learning needs, review their performance or that of the practice organisation, and reflect on what improvements to make. You might want to do a selection of the reflection exercises, or all of them. Alternatively, you might have other ideas for exercises to identify your learning needs or gaps in the practice team performance. The main objective is to reflect on what you have learned and to apply that learning in practice both as an individual and with work colleagues.

You should transfer information from these needs assessment exercises to the relevant slots in your personal development plan, or to your practice personal and professional development plan if you are working as a team. Adopt a wide-based approach to improving quality – think of how you are establishing a clinical governance culture in your own practice team through your timed action plans.

What should you do next?

Study the templates for a personal development plan on pages 141–151 or a practice personal and professional development plan on pages 165–172. You will be filling these in as you go along. Decide whether you will be starting out on your personal development plan or working with colleagues on the practice learning plan. Everyone's personal development plans should mesh with the practice learning plan by the time you have finished drawing them up.

Make changes as a result – to your workplace, or to the equipment in your practice, or to the advice you give patients, or to the way in which you prevent and manage overweight and obesity and the various complicating problems associated with them.

References

1 Wakley G, Chambers R and Field S (2000) *Continuing Professional Development: making it happen.* Radcliffe Medical Press, Oxford.
2 Chambers R and Wakley G (2000) *Making Clinical Governance Work for You.* Radcliffe Medical Press, Oxford.
3 National Audit Office (2001) *Tackling Obesity in England.* The Stationery Office, London.
4 World Health Organization (1998) *Obesity: preventing and managing the global epidemic. Report of WHO Consultation on Obesity.* World Health Organization, Geneva.

CHAPTER 1

The scale of the problem: overweight and obesity

Definitions

Overweight and obesity are most commonly defined by clinicians in terms of the *body mass index* (BMI).

$$\text{BMI} = \frac{\text{weight in kilogrammes}}{(\text{height in metres})^2}.$$

Overweight is usually defined as a BMI of between 25 and 29.9, and obesity as a BMI of 30 or over (*see* Table 1.1).

Table 1.1 Classification and risk of overweight in adults according to BMI[1,2]

Classification	BMI (kg/m²)	Risk of comorbidities
Underweight	< 18.5	Low (but risk of other clinical problems increased, and may be secondary to serious illness)
Desirable range	18.5–24.9	Average
Overweight	25.0–29.9	Increased
Obese class I	30.0–34.9	Moderate
Obese class II	35.0–39.9	Severe
Obese class III (also known as 'morbid' or 'severe' obesity)	⩾ 40.0	Very severe

Body mass index does not distinguish between mass due to body fat and muscles, nor does it take into account the distribution of fat around the body. Some individuals who might not be defined as obese according to their BMIs may still have a high degree of abdominal obesity (also termed 'central' obesity). Central obesity is measured by the waist

Table 1.2 Waist circumferences that denote increased risk of metabolic complications of obesity in Caucasian people[1]

	Risk of complications	
	Increased	Substantially increased
Men	>94 cm (~37 in)	>102 cm (~40 in)
Women	>80 cm (~32 in)	>88 cm (~35 in)

circumference or the waist:hip ratio. The relative distribution of fat between the waist and hip predicts subsequent coronary artery disease better than body mass index. There are increased health risks from obesity when the waist circumference exceeds 94 cm for men and 80 cm for women.[2] Table 1.2 gives more information about the extent of health risks associated with central obesity.

Health experts have called for primary care clinicians to record the waist circumference of patients as well as their BMI, and to tailor interventions such as weight reduction and the primary and secondary prevention of cardiovascular disease according to abdominal fat measurements rather than the BMI. However, this is still infrequent practice.[3]

Prevalence of obesity[1,4–6]

The prevalence of obesity throughout Europe has increased sharply over the last 20 years, second only to that in the USA, and closely followed by many developing nations in Asia. In the majority of European countries the prevalence of obesity increased by 10–40% between 1980 and the late 1990s. Current rates of obesity in European countries are in the range 10–20% for men, and 10–25% for women.

The UK has the fastest growing rate of obesity in Europe, which has almost trebled in the past 20 years. Box 1.1 gives the figures for England.

Box 1.1 Prevalence rates of overweight and obesity in England[1,4,5]

Increase in the prevalence of:	*1980*	*1997*
Adult males who are overweight	39%	62%
Adult females who are overweight	32%	53%
Adult males who are obese	6%	17%
Adult females who are obese	8%	20%

overweight, BMI = 25–29.9; obese, BMI $\geqslant$ 30.

There is a similar prevalence of obesity in England, Wales and Scotland. In Scotland, 44% of men are overweight and a further 14% are obese, and 32% of women are overweight and a further 17% are obese. Overall, around 1% of the adult population in the UK has severe obesity with a BMI of $\geqslant$ 40.

Table 1.3 demonstrates how much more common obesity is in England and the USA compared with other countries.

The increasing incidence of obesity and overweight in children is of equal concern, where the rate of increase mirrors that in adults.[7] A recent study in the UK looking at children under 5 years of age showed a significant increase in childhood obesity in the 10 years between 1989 and 1998. There was a 60% increase in the prevalence of overweight (defined as BMI above the 85th centile) and a 70% increase in the prevalence of obesity (defined as BMI above the 95th centile) among children aged 3 to 4 years. The figures showed that the proportion of children who were overweight increased from 15% in 1989 to 24% in 1998, and for obese children the figure rose from 5% to 9%.[8]

Even if obesity continues at current rates, and the increasing prevalence is halted, half of those adolescents who are obese with a BMI greater than the 95th percentile will go on to become obese adults.

Table 1.3 Prevalence (%) of obesity (BMI >30) in representative samples of men and women from various countries[1,4]

Country	*Year*	*Age range (years)*	*Men (%)*	*Women (%)*
England	1996	16–64	16.0	17.0
The Netherlands	1995	20–59	8.4	8.3
USA	1991	20–74	19.7	24.7
Japan	1993	$\geqslant$ 20	1.8	2.6

The number of people with diabetes is expected to double by 2010 – due to obesity. Therefore obesity will reduce the likelihood of effectively combating heart disease and other conditions associated with obesity, such as cancer, arthritic pain, respiratory and gastrointestinal complaints. Type 2 diabetes is now seen in American children and is expected in UK children, too, if childhood trends towards obesity continue.

One in five members of the adult population is obese – representing around 250 of the average general practitioner's patient list. Around 1% of adult patients will be morbidly obese – equivalent to 70 individuals in a practice with an adult patient population of 7000.

Overweight and obese people are at a considerable social disadvantage because of the stereotypical images society has created. They may be at a disadvantage in relation to their slimmer peers when they apply for jobs, and they may also have a poor self-image and unsatisfactory personal relationships.

Causes of obesity

The causes of overweight and obesity are complex and multifactorial. An individual who maintains their weight over time is in a state of 'energy balance' – that is, the total energy taken in through food is equalled by the total energy expended through activity and metabolism. Obesity occurs when a person is in 'positive energy balance' – that is, when energy intake exceeds energy output. The reasons why this positive energy balance comes about are greatly influenced by genetic predisposition, behavioural patterns and cultural influences.

Energy intake – energy expenditure = change in body fat stores[4]

In the UK it is generally held that we consume on average less calories per day than we did a generation ago, and that it is the significant reduction in physical activity levels among the UK adult and child populations which is the crucial factor in triggering obesity. However, when data were collected in the 1970s, calorific intake was calculated from the amount of food identified as having been consumed at home. The data excluded the consumption of alcoholic drinks and food purchased and consumed outside the home (e.g. at work, in snack bars or in restaurants), all of which have increased significantly during the past 20 years. This omission is important, as there has been a cultural shift towards less regular eating habits and the consumption of

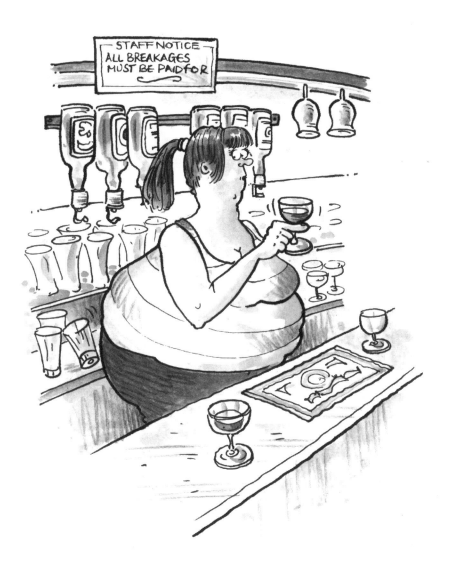

more snack meals at home and at work.[5] Thus it is likely that it is both eating too much and engaging in too little physical activity that accounts for the rising trends towards overweight and obesity.

The incidence of obesity increases with age, and the wide variety of causes and associations are listed in Box 1.2.[9]

Box 1.2 Variety of causes of obesity and associations with health conditions[9]

Too little physical activity
Sedentary lifestyle (e.g. watching too much television).

Surplus calorie and fat intake
Changes in dietary behaviour (e.g. eating fast foods, excess alcohol intake).

Environmental factors
Overweight and obesity are more prevalent in lower socio-economic classes. Lifestyle is important – obesity may run in families without there being a genetic cause.

Genetic factors
Twin studies have shown a genetic link related to low metabolic rate and energy efficiency. Laurence–Moon–Biedl's syndrome and Prader-Willi's syndrome are examples of genetic causes of obesity.

Psychological factors
Disturbance of self-image, including some eating disorders (e.g. bulimia), and depression.

Endocrine factors
Corticosteroid excess, hypothyroidism, hypothalamic malfunction, pituitary disease and polycystic ovaries.

Developmental factors
Hypertrophic obesity (increased size of fat cells is usual in adult-onset obesity) and hyperplastic obesity (increased number of fat cells is usual in juvenile-onset obesity) are now thought to coexist. Obesity is more common with increasing age.

Drugs
Side-effects of drugs such as corticosteroids, insulin, sulphonyl-ureas and lithium.

Influence of social class

Obesity and overweight are more prevalent in lower socio-economic groups. The BMI of women in manual classes tends to be higher than that of women in non-manual classes. This trend is less consistent for men because of the extent of physical activity by those employed in manual labour. The prevalence of obesity in women in social class I is 12%, compared with 21% in social class V. Around 10% of men in social class I and 13% of men in social class V are obese.[1,10]

The prevalence of obesity in women who change social class as they grow older tends to be that for the class which they join.[4]

Level of education

The highest prevalence of obesity was found among less well-qualified individuals in one national study in the UK. Around 11% of less well-educated men aged 43 years with qualifications up to and including O-levels had a BMI of 30, compared with only 5% of men with degree qualifications. For women, the corresponding figures were 15% and 4%, respectively.[4]

Ethnicity

The likelihood of obesity varies between different ethnic groups. South Asians living in the UK are at greater risk of developing central obesity than African-Caribbeans and Caucasians. Compared with women in general, black Caribbean women living in England are twice as likely to have 'morbid' obesity according to a recent health survey.[11] It has been reported that 32% of black Caribbean women are obese (BMI $\geqslant 30\,\text{kg/m}^2$), compared with Indian women (20% of whom are obese), Pakistani women (26%), Bangladeshi women (10%), Chinese women (5%), Irish women (21%) and women in the general population (21%).[11]

In men, rates of obesity vary with different ethnic characteristics, too. Around 18% of black Caribbean men living in the UK are obese, compared with 12% of Indian men, 13% of Pakistani men, 5% of Bangladeshi men, 6% of Chinese men, 20% of Irish men and 19% of men in the general population who are obese.[11]

> **Box 1.3** Ethnic differences in self-perception of obesity
>
> There seems to be less self-awareness and perception of obesity among South Asian women living in the UK compared with European women. The study was based on the assumption that people were more likely to lose weight if they perceived themselves to be overweight or obese. The researchers found that ethnic differences persisted even among those with diabetes, who they had expected to have a more realistic body weight perception as a result of diabetes education.[12]

Levels of physical inactivity

The general population's level of activity – or rather *inactivity* – has plummeted during the last few decades. Employment and leisure activities have become much more sedentary, and use of private cars has increased. It is estimated that 50 years ago each British adult expended energy equivalent to running a marathon race every week, due to the active nature of their work and domestic tasks. The average person in England now watches over 26 hours of television a week, compared with 13 hours in the 1960s. Children spend many hours watching videos and playing with computer games rather than playing active games.[13]

This decrease in energy expenditure has not been matched by a sufficient decrease in calorific intake. Physical inactivity doubles the risk of coronary heart disease, is a major risk factor for stroke, and contributes to the increased frequency of overweight and obesity. There is a graded inverse relationship between physical activity and the risk of coronary events occurring.

Among the general UK population, only one-third of men (33%) and one-fifth of women (21%) meet the current guidelines for physical activity – that is moderate or vigorous activity for at least 30 minutes at a time, on five or more days a week. Pakistani and Bangladeshi women living in England are between three and four times more likely to take part in vigorous activity compared with the general female population, whereas Indian and black Caribbean women are considerably less likely to do so. Black Caribbean men had the highest levels of participation in physical activity but ethnic differences are less marked for men than for women.[11]

The commonest types of physical activity for men are sports and exercise, and heavy housework. For women, heavy housework is by far the most frequently reported type of physical activity, followed by sports and exercise.[11]

Metabolism and energy expenditure

The main components of energy expenditure are basal metabolic rate, thermogenesis and physical activity. Thermogenesis includes the following:

- any heat production that is required to maintain body temperature
- heat loss associated with the absorption, metabolism and transport of ingested food
- heat production to dissipate excess dietary energy.

In sedentary people the relative proportions are 60–75% expended as the basal metabolism, 10% for thermogenesis and 25% for physical activity. In sedentary people the basal metabolic rate is about 5–10% higher than the minimum rate which occurs whilst asleep. The basal metabolic rate is higher in overweight and obese people than in people of 'ideal' weight, as weight gain increases the size of muscle and visceral organs as well as fat. There is no evidence that obese people have extraordinarily low basal metabolic rates that account for their obesity.[4]

Appetite control and neurotransmission

Different regulatory mechanisms exert physiological control over appetite, hunger and satiation. Social and environmental influences can overpower these physiological mechanisms.

Several neurotransmitters are involved in the regulation of food intake. The role of dopamine in obesity is poorly understood. Drugs that block dopamine D_s receptors increase appetite and result in significant weight gain, whereas drugs that increase the dopamine concentration in the brain are anorexigenic. There is speculation that dopamine deficiency in obese people perpetuates their pathological eating and renders them more susceptible to addictive behaviours, including compulsive food intake.[14]

Hyperplastic versus hypertrophic adipose cells

Increased deposition of fat is normally accommodated by expansion (hypertrophy) or contraction of existing fat cells. This is a reversible process that occurs with varying daily intake. When the existing fat cells are full, more fat cells are created (hyperplasia). Once formed, these new fat cells are irreversible or at least remain for years. There is speculation that a large number of fat cells may predispose a person to gain fat easily and become obese. It may be that there are factors which induce hyperplasia other than the state of fullness of existing fat cells. If we understood these factors, we might be able to influence them.[4]

Genetics

There is a strong genetic influence on obesity and the distribution of fat tissue. Obesity is regarded as a group of heterogeneous disorders rather than a single-gene disorder. Genetic influences seem to account for 50–70% of the difference in BMI in later life in both monozygotic and dizygotic twins reared apart.[4] Studies of adopted children have shown a strong relationship between the BMI of the biological parents and the adoptee for BMIs ranging from very thin to very fat, but little relationship between the adoptive parents and the adoptee.[4]

However, the rapid increase in the prevalence of obesity in developed countries indicates the powerful influence of the environment, as opposed to genetic causes.

Low levels of physical activity may be a familial trait which predisposes to obesity.

Psychological factors

The behavioural and other psychological conditions that are associated with obesity can have genetic or environmental origins. It is difficult to differentiate between psychological factors that are causes and effects in accounting for obesity in an individual or their response to treatment.

For instance, a 'binge-eating' pattern may be present in 20–30% of people who are obese. Binge eating is 'eating in a discrete period of time, an amount of food that is larger than most people would eat in a similar period under similar circumstances'. It involves a 'sense of a lack of control during that episode, feeling unable to stop eating or control what or how much to eat'.[15] Binge eating is linked with emotional distress. There are higher levels of personality disorders and depressive disorders among obese 'binge eaters' than among non-obese 'binge eaters'. It is uncertain whether the 'binge eating' precedes the depression or arises as a result of the eating disorder.[4]

Comorbidity

People with a BMI of 25 or above have an increased risk of developing comorbidities, which is further increased with BMI values of 30 or more. Virtually all obese people will have developed physical symptoms by 40 years of age, and the majority will require medical intervention for diseases that develop as a direct result of their obesity by the age of 60 years. For BMI values of 40 or more (severe or morbid obesity), the risk of a life-threatening disease developing as a direct result of obesity is extremely high.

Obesity not only causes much psychological morbidity, but is also a primary risk factor in the development of hypertension, cardiovascular disease, stroke, diabetes mellitus, hyperlipidaemia, osteoarthritis, and cancer of the breast, ovary, prostate and colon.

Obesity is associated with a considerably increased risk of endometrial cancer (the relative risk is 5.4 for those weighing 40% or more than average[16]), and a greater risk of breast cancer in premenopausal women, and to some extent of bowel cancer in men.

The proportion of common diseases that can be attributed to excess body weight is shown in Table 1.4. Hip fracture is expressed as a negative proportion, as people who are excessively overweight or obese are less likely to experience a hip fracture than those who are underweight.

Table 1.4 Proportion of various diseases that are attributable to excess weight $(BMI > 27 \, kg/m^2)^1$

Disease	Proportion (%)
Obesity	100.0
Hypertension	24.1
Myocardial infarction	13.9
Angina pectoris	20.5
Stroke	25.8
Venous thrombosis	7.7
Type 2 diabetes	24.1
Hyperlipidaemia	7.7
Gout	20.0
Osteoarthritis	11.8
Gall-bladder disease	14.3
Colorectal cancer	4.7
Breast cancer	3.2
Genitourinary cancer	9.1
Hip fracture	−3.5

Obesity leads to premature mortality. A man weighing more than 140% of the average weight is 5.2 times more likely to die of diabetes than a man of ideal weight. Similarly, women who are more than 140% overweight are 7.9 times more likely to die of diabetes than women of ideal weight. After adjustment for age and smoking, the risk of a fatal or non-fatal myocardial infarction among women with a BMI greater than 29 is three times that among lean women.[1]

Osteoarthritis is a common complication of obesity, especially in weight-bearing joints such as the knees and hips. The risk of osteoarthritis is related to the total amount of fat, rather than to the extent of abdominal fat.

People who are obese are more likely to develop gallstones because of their higher output of cholesterol in bile.

Obesity is also associated with reproductive and menstrual disorders.

Sleep apnoea is caused by the physical pressure effects of fat on the chest wall and upward pushing on the liver, which compresses the lungs and leads to poor lung ventilation. In addition, fat around the neck of an obese person may compress the trachea.[1]

Box 1.4 Resistin links obesity with type 2 diabetes[17]

A newly identified hormone, resistin, links obesity to type 2 diabetes and partly explains how obesity predisposes people to diabetes. Resistin is thought to be secreted by fat cells and then to modify the body's sensitivity to insulin, causing insulin resistance.

The public health approach to obesity as a chronic disease

The Disability Adjusted Life Year (DALY) is a measure devised by the World Bank that estimates the size of a health problem in an area, based on death and disability.[18] The complex method of calculation takes into account the number of years lost due to early death and the estimated time lived with the disability for an individual disease or health problem. For some problems, such as cancer, the main component of the DALY comes from the premature mortality, whereas for a health problem such as mental illness, the major component of the disease burden comes from disability.

The DALY can help health planners to compare population needs arising from different diseases or health problems. It can help to

Table 1.5 Disease burden in South Staffordshire that is attributable to major risk factors[18]

Risk factor	Proportion of DALYs
Alcohol consumption	5.4%
Smoking	4.4%
Relative poverty	3.9%
Low vegetable/fruit content of diet	3.2%
Occupational risks	3.1%
Obesity	3.1%
Drug addiction	2.6%
Diet high in saturated fat	1.8%
Unemployment	1.5%
Physical inactivity	1.4%

prioritise the investment of resources in tackling the health problems of a local area (e.g. with the health improvement programme), or at a national level.

The measure can also be used to estimate the importance of various determinants of health or risk factors for disease. Table 1.5 summarises the DALYs that are attributable to the major risk factors calculated for one health district of England, showing obesity as accounting for a higher proportion of death and disability than physical inactivity, but being less important than alcohol, smoking and deprivation.

Box 1.5

In 1995 a leading public health physician wrote:

Overweight and obesity have an underestimated impact on public health and therefore on national economic costs . . . . The needed transformation in thinking on transport, environment, work facilities, education, health and food policies and perhaps in social and economic policies is unlikely when governments are wedded to individualism, but without these changes to enhance physical activity and alter food quality, societies are doomed to escalating obesity rates.[19]

The changes in health, social and transport policies that have been published and implemented in the UK since 1995 have made a good start in tackling obesity – but there is still a long way to go before obesity levels even start to level off.

Reflection exercises

Exercise 1

Undertake a 'Strengths, Weaknesses, Opportunities and Threats' (SWOT) analysis of your practice's approach to the management of patients who are overweight or obese.

Look at the general philosophy of the practice team. Do they regard obesity as a serious health issue? Are staff up to date about what constitute effective interventions for weight management? Do you have a practice protocol for the management of children and adults who are overweight or obese? If so, do practice staff adhere to the practice protocol consistently? Do you have access to a community dietitian or a psychologist with an interest in eating disorders and obesity?

You can undertake a SWOT analysis of your own performance or that of your practice team or practice organisation, working it out either on your own, or with a workmate or mentor, or with a group of colleagues. Brainstorm the strengths, weaknesses, opportunities and threats of the situation.

The strengths and weaknesses of individual practitioners might include knowledge, experience, expertise, decision making, communication skills, interprofessional relationships, political skills, time-keeping, organisational skills, teaching skills and research skills. The strengths and weaknesses of the practice organisation might relate to most of these aspects, too, as well as resources (staff, skills, structural).

Opportunities might relate to unexploited potential strengths, expected changes, options for career development pathways, and hobbies and interests that might usefully be expanded.

Threats will include factors and circumstances that prevent you from achieving your aims with regard to personal, professional and practice development.

Prioritise the important factors. Draw up goals and a timed action plan to overcome gaps or weaknesses and make the most of the opportunities.

Exercise 2

Look at your practice population's health needs and see what you may need to learn as an individual or as a practice team in order to address those needs more effectively. Review the numbers of patients who are overweight or obese and their exercise habits. How current are the details recorded in their medical notes or computerised records? (If you cannot set up an audit on your computer to look at the date of record entry, either obtain this information from the paper records, or simply check whether or not you have ever made a record of BMI.)

Create a detailed profile of your practice population. Ask your primary care organisation (PCO) or the local public health department for information about your practice population and comparative information about the general population living in the district. This would include morbidity and mortality statistics, referral patterns, age/sex mix, ethnicity, and population trends.

Include information about the wider determinants of health, such as housing, numbers in and types of employment, geographical location, the environment, crime and safety, educational attainment and socio-economic data. Focus on the current state of health inequalities within your practice population, or between your practice population and the district as a whole.

You as an individual or as a practice team might learn more about the causes of morbidity and mortality in your population so that you can institute a more effective preventative approach. Focus on areas where you can make changes in people's behaviour or health status (e.g. weight management), rather than on topics that are beyond your direct control (e.g. improving the transport system).

This practice population profile will help you to prioritise your learning and target service development at the health needs of your patients. This mapping process will enable you to appreciate the overlap of overweight and obesity with the other medical conditions with which they are associated. You could combine learning about the management of obesity with coronary heart disease or diabetes for example.

Now that you have completed these interactive reflection exercises, transfer the information to the empty template of the personal development plan on pages 141–151 if you are working on your own learning plan, or to the practice personal and professional development plan on pages 165–172 if you are working on a practice team learning plan. Don't forget to keep the evidence of your learning in your personal portfolio.

References

1 Garrow J and Summerbell C (2002) Obesity. In: *Health Care Needs Assessment*. Third Series. Radcliffe Medical Press, Oxford.

2 World Health Organization (1997) *Obesity: preventing and managing the global epidemic.* World Health Organization, Geneva.

3 Despres JP, Lemieux I and Prud'homme D (2001) Treatment of obesity: need to focus on high risk abdominally obese patients. *BMJ.* **322**: 716–20.

4 Garrow J (chair) (1999) *Obesity. Report of the British Nutrition Foundation Task Force.* Blackwell Science, Oxford.

5 National Audit Office (2001) *Tackling Obesity in England.* National Audit Office, London.

6 Scottish Intercollegiate Guidelines Network (SIGN) (1996) *Obesity in Scotland: integrating prevention with weight management.* SIGN, Edinburgh.

7 Chinn S and Rona RJ (1994) Trends in weight for height and triceps skinfold thickness for English and Scottish children, 1972–1982 and 1982–1990. *Paediatr Perinat Epidemiol.* **8**: 90–106.

8 Bundred P, Kitchiner D and Buchan I (2000) Prevalence of overweight and obese children between 1989 and 1998: population-based series of cross-sectional studies. *BMJ.* **320**: 326–8.

9 Campbell I (2001) Primary care guidelines aim to simplify obesity management. *Guidelines Pract.* **4**: 69–74.

10 NHS Centre for Reviews and Dissemination (1997) The prevention and treatment of obesity. *Effect Health Care Bull.* **3**: 1–12.

11 Erens B, Primatesta P and Prior G (eds) (2001) *Health Survey for England. The health of minority ethnic groups '99.* The Stationery Office, London.

12 Patel S, Bhopal R, Unwin N *et al.* (2001) Mismatch between perceived and actual overweight in diabetic and non-diabetic populations: a comparative study of South Asian and European women. *J Epidemiol Commun Health.* **55**: 332–3.

13 Prentice A and Jebb S (1995) Obesity in Britain: gluttony or sloth? *BMJ.* **311**: 437–9.

14 Wang GJ, Volkow N, Logan J *et al.* (2001) Brain dopamine and obesity. *Lancet.* **357**: 354–7.

15 Waller D (2001) Binge eating. *BMJ.* **322**: 343.

16 Cummings J and Bingham S (1998) Diet and the prevention of cancer. *BMJ.* **317**: 1636–40.

17 Berger A (2001) Resistin: a new hormone that links obesity with type 2 diabetes. *BMJ.* **322**: 293.

18 Wall M (1999) *Melting the Iceberg: changing the burden of disease in South Staffordshire.* The Annual Report of the Director of Public Health. South Staffordshire Health Authority, Stafford.

19 James W (1995) A public health approach to the problem of obesity. *Int J Obesity.* **19 (Supplement 3)**: S37–45.

CHAPTER 2

Clinical governance and the management of overweight and obesity

Clinical governance is about doing anything and everything required to maximise the quality of healthcare or services provided for, and received by, individual patients or the general population – in this case, those who are overweight or obese.[1,2]

We should be able to use clinical governance to improve the detection and control of chronic conditions such as obesity. Clinical governance is inclusive, making quality everyone's business, whether they are a doctor, a nurse or other health professional, a manager, a member of staff or a strategic planner. Good healthcare relies on the multidisciplinary team to support the overweight or obese person in self-managing their condition, inasmuch as they are able to do so. Delivering best practice requires sufficient clinical staff who are up to date and relate well to their patients, working with efficient systems and procedures that are patient friendly.

Components of clinical governance[2]

The components of clinical governance are not new. However, bringing them together under the banner of clinical governance and introducing more explicit accountability for performance is a new style of working.

The following 14 themes are core components of professional and service development which together form a comprehensive approach to providing high-quality healthcare services and clinical governance.[2] These are illustrated in Figure 2.1.

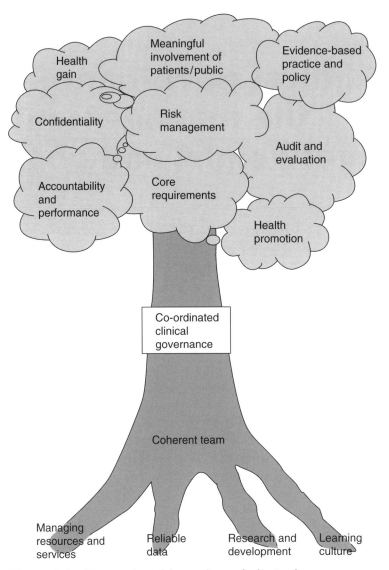

Figure 2.1: 'Routes' and branches of clinical governance.

If you interweave these 14 components into your individual and workplace-based personal and professional development plans you will have addressed the requirements for clinical governance at the same time.

1 *Learning culture*: for patients and staff in the practice or primary care organisation, or in secondary care.
2 *Research and development culture*: in the practice or throughout the health service.

3 *Reliable and accurate data*: in the practice, and across the primary care organisation and the NHS as a seamless whole.

4 *Well-managed resources and services*: as individuals, as a practice, across the NHS and in conjunction with other organisations.

5 *Coherent team*: well-integrated teams within a practice, including attached staff.

6 *Meaningful involvement of patients and the public*: including those with obesity, their families and the general population.

7 *Health gain*: from improving the health of staff and patients in a practice, between practices and within a primary care organisation.

8 *Confidentiality*: of information at the reception desk, in consultations, in medical notes, between practitioners and with the outside world.

9 *Evidence-based practice and policy*: applying it in everyday practice, in the district and across the NHS.

10 *Accountability and performance*: for standards, performance of individuals and the practice, both to the public and to those in authority.

11 *Core requirements*: good fit with skill mix and whether individuals are competent to do their jobs; communication, workforce numbers and morale at practice level.

12 *Health promotion*: for patients, the public, your staff and colleagues – both opportunistic and in general, or targeting those who are obese.

13 *Audit and evaluation*: for instance, of the extent to which individuals and practice teams adhere to best practice in the management of overweight and obesity.

14 *Risk management*: being competent to detect those at risk, and reducing the risks and probabilities of ill health. Risk management is really important at all stages in the management of obesity, including detection, weight control and prevention of relapse.

The challenges to delivering clinical governance

Delivering high-quality healthcare with guaranteed minimum standards of care at all times is a major challenge. At present, the quality of healthcare is patchy and variable. We are not very good at detecting under-performance and rectifying it at an early stage. The small number of clinicians who do under-perform exert a disproportionately large effect on the public's confidence. Causes of under-performance in an individual might be a result of a lack of knowledge or skills, poor attitudes, ill health or a lack of resources. Poor management is nearly always a contributory reason for inadequate clinical services.

We need to understand why variation exists and explore ways of reducing inequalities. Variation in the quality of healthcare provided is common – between different practices in the same locality, between staff of the same discipline working in the same practice or unit, and between care given to some groups of the population rather than others.

Clinical governance offers a co-ordinated approach to overcoming these areas of risk.[3] The complex cultural change that will be required to deliver uniformly excellent care is immense. We need to develop measurable outcomes that professionals, patients and the public consider to be relevant and meaningful. Then we can assess the progress made through implementing clinical governance in the targets you set out in your action plans.

Learning culture

Education and training programmes should be relevant to service needs, whether at organisational or individual levels. Continuing professional development (CPD) programmes need to meet both the learning needs of individual health professionals and the wider service development needs of the NHS. You should no longer opt for CPD activities according to what you *want* to do, but rather according to what you *need* to do. Clinical governance underpins professional and service development.

Box 2.1

Individual personal development plans
will feed into a
**workplace or practice-based personal and
professional development plan**
that will feed into
the primary care organisation's business plan
all of which are
underpinned by clinical governance.[4]

Multidisciplinary learning helps the team to work closely together to provide well-co-ordinated multidisciplinary care.

Applying research and development in practice

The findings of the many thousands of research papers providing evidence about the management of obesity that are published in reputable journals each year are rarely applied in practice by health professionals. This is because few health professionals or managers read such journals regularly, and therefore they are unaware of the research findings. Most practice teams do not have a system for reviewing important research papers and translating that review into practical action. The primary care organisation might help by feeding important new evidence to its constituent practices or the general public. Agreeing on local disease templates (e.g. for the management of obesity or coronary heart disease) backed by resources should enable change to happen.

Box 2.2 Reducing dietary fat decreases cardiovascular risk[5]

Less total fat or less of any individual fatty acid fraction in the diet is beneficial. A reduction of over 20% in total serum cholesterol concentration can result in a corresponding 25% decrease in mortality from coronary heart disease.

A recent systematic review of trials that modified or reduced fat intake for at least six months has concluded that there is a 'small but potentially important reduction in cardiovascular risk with reduction or modification of dietary fat intake, seen particularly in trials of longer duration'. There were reductions in cardiovascular events of up to 24% in trials lasting for at least two years. However, it was not clear whether it was the duration of the intervention or the length of follow-up that was critical in determining whether the intervention was effective. Yet there was little effect on total mortality.

Incorporation of research-based evidence into everyday practice should promote policies on effective working, improve quality and contribute to a clinical governance culture.

A number of research trials conducted on obese people with hypertension have demonstrated that small losses of weight, such as 2 to 5 kg, reduce mean blood pressure by 10–13 mmHg when the lower weight is maintained over the long term.[6]

Box 2.3 Losing weight reduces blood pressure[7]

There is now consistent evidence that weight loss reduces blood pressure not only in people who are overweight and hypertensive, but also in those who are overweight with high–normal blood pressure.

In one study of 1200 people whose BMI values were between 25 and 37, none of whom were being treated for hypertension, those who had lost at least 4.5 kg of weight by six months showed an initial average fall in systolic and diastolic blood pressures of 8 or 9 mmHg, which was maintained at 36 months follow-up. The lower levels of blood pressure at six months were not maintained at follow-up in those who failed to maintain the weight loss of 4.5 kg or more at six months.

Reliable and accurate data

Clinicians, patients and administrators need access to reliable and accurate data. Set the following standards for a general practice.

- Keep records in chronological order.
- Summarise medical records, within a specified time period for records of new patients.
- Review dates for checks on medication, with audit in place to monitor whether standards are adhered to, and to plan for under-performance if necessary.
- Use computers for diagnostic recording, and agree Read codes for classifying weight and other lifestyle factors.
- Record information from external sources (e.g. hospital, other organisations) that is relevant to individual patients or the practice.

Box 2.4

Read coding (Clinical Terms Version 3) will be amalgamated with the system used by the College of American Pathologists to create a new coding system called SNOMED* clinical terms. It is expected that this new system will be available in late 2001 and will eventually replace the Read coding system. Any future transfer will be easier if medical records are already well ordered and classified.

* Systematized Nomenclature of Medicine.

Keep good written records of policies and audits that relate to patients' body mass indices. An inspection at any time should show what audits have been undertaken and when, the changes in practice organisation that followed, the extent of staff training undertaken, and the future programme of monitoring.

The government wants to create an electronic health record (EHR) by 2005. This is a lifelong record giving details of a patient's health and healthcare. Pilots of EHRs are considering the ethical and operational issues.

Well-managed resources and services

The things you need to achieve best practice should be in the right place at the right time and working correctly every time.

Set standards in your practice or workplace for the following:

- access to premises and availability of services for people with special needs (e.g. those with disability due to heart disease or stroke)
- provision of routine and urgent appointments (e.g. for those with coronary heart disease)
- access to and provision for referral for investigation or treatment
- pro-active monitoring of chronic illness and disability
- alternatives to face-to-face consultations
- consultation length.

The primary care services to which the public requires access include information, advice, triage and treatment, continuity of care, personal care, emergency care and other services.

Systems should be designed to prevent and detect errors. Therefore keep systems simple and sensible, and inform everyone how those systems operate so that they are less likely to bypass a system or make errors. Establish good systems for the follow-up of patients who have sought help for their obesity. For example, flag those patients' notes on the computer so that next time they consult you can monitor their weight and reinforce lifestyle advice. Undertake an audit at intervals in order to monitor their progress.

Box 2.5

Obesity is thought to cost the UK over £2 billion each year at current prices. If nothing is done about the problem, then by 2010 it may be costing us twice this amount.[8]

Coherent teamwork

Teams do produce better patient care than single practitioners operating in a fragmented way. Effective teams make the most of the different contributions of individual clinical disciplines in delivering patient care. The characteristics of effective teams are as follows:

- shared ownership of a common purpose
- clear goals for the contributions that each discipline makes
- open communication between team members
- opportunities for team members to enhance their skills.

A team approach helps different team members to adopt an evidence-based approach to patient care – by having to justify their approach to the rest of the team.[9] The disciplines necessary for providing team-based care for patients who want help for their obesity include the GP and practice nurse, other community nurses such as health visitors and midwives, non-clinical staff, and the dietitian, community pharmacist and psychologist.

Meaningful involvement of patients and the public

Patients or carers, non-users of services, the local community, particular subgroups of the population or the general public will all have useful feedback and views. For example, ask for their views about the quality or type of healthcare on offer, planning of future services, your systems, or how to locate services closer to the patient.

The aims of user involvement and public participation include better outcomes of individual care, better health of the population, more locally responsive services and greater ownership of health services. Those planning the services should develop a better understanding of why and how local services need to be changed.[10] Consumers and other lay people representing a wide variety of private and public sector interests include specialist voluntary bodies such as the Association for the Study of Obesity, the private-sector slimming industry, employers, sports promoters, etc.

Box 2.6

Peer education is at the heart of a community development approach in one project within Leicester Health Action Zone. Trained voluntary peer educators are working with the local population to promote good diet and exercise as part of an initiative to prevent coronary heart disease and diabetes. In total, 78% of the local population are of Bangladeshi, Indian or Pakistani origin. Other volunteers lead chair-based exercise sessions for housebound people.

Health gain

The two general approaches to improving health are the 'population' approach, which focuses on measures to improve health through the community, and the 'high-risk' approach, which focuses on vulnerable individuals who are at high risk of the condition or hazard.

The population strategy aims to shift the whole distribution of a risk factor in a favourable direction. However, the 'prevention paradox' means that preventive actions that greatly benefit the population at large may bring only small benefits for individuals.[11] A population-based approach must target the whole population, from young people to older adults, through educational programmes that promote caloric balance through exercise and sensible diet.

Box 2.7

Changing the population distribution of a risk factor is more effective overall than targeting people who are at high risk. At a population level, greater relative health gain can be expected if sedentary people take up moderate activity than if those who are already active take up more vigorous activity. It is thought that a 10% reduction in saturated fat intake among the UK population would reduce deaths from coronary heart disease by 20–30%.[12]

The high-risk approach aims to detect people at high risk of disease and to lower their risk by treatment. We generally use a targeted approach in primary care to identify people who are at risk, rather than a population-based approach.

The two approaches are not mutually exclusive, and they often need to be combined with legislation and community action. Health goals include the following:

- a good quality of life
- avoiding premature death
- equal opportunities for health.

Local strategies to address obesity include encouraging the local population to increase the extent of their physical activity and adopt a healthy diet. Policies on promoting active transport (e.g. walking and cycling) instead of the car, and promoting active recreation in society, are being tried. There are special initiatives targeting children and young people to ensure that they receive education on health, diet and physical activity, and that the school environment promotes healthy lifestyles and physical recreation. The National Audit Office report[8] suggests that a realistic five-year aim for a district might be to keep the local prevalence of obesity constant, rather than to set unachievable targets to reduce the prevalence.

Box 2.8

General practice management of obesity consists of three approaches:[8]

- general advice to those consulting, as well as personal advice about weight control, diet and physical exercise for individual patients
- personal advice about lifestyle change and weight loss, supported by prescribed drug therapy
- referral to a weight-loss specialist, possibly involving drug therapy or even surgery.

Confidentiality

Confidentiality is a component of clinical governance that is often overlooked. Experienced health professionals and managers may assume that junior or new staff know all about confidentiality, and of course they may not. There are many difficult situations in the NHS where one person asks for information about another individual's medical condition. For example, it is not always clear-cut whether test results should be given to or withheld from someone else enquiring on the patient's behalf if the patient is vulnerable in some way (e.g. affected by a severe stroke).

The Caldicott Committee Report describes the following principles of good practice to safeguard confidentiality when information is being used for non-clinical purposes.[13]

- Justify the purpose.
- Do not use patient-identifiable information unless it is absolutely necessary to do so.
- Use the minimum necessary patient-identifiable information.
- Access to patient-identifiable information should be on a strict need-to-know basis.
- Everyone with access to patient-identifiable information should be aware of his or her responsibilities.

Evidence-based culture: policy and practice

The key features that determined whether or not local guidelines worked in one initiative[14] were as follows.

- There was multidisciplinary involvement in drawing them up.
- A systematic review of the literature underpinned the guidelines, with graded recommendations for best practice linked to the evidence.
- There was ownership at national and local levels.
- A local implementation plan ensured that the needs for resources, time, staff, education and training were foreseen, met and supported.
- Plans were made to sustain the guidelines – which were user friendly and could be modified to suit individual practitioners and patients.

There are several systems of grading evidence. One classification[15] that is often quoted gives the strength of evidence as shown in Box 2.9.

Box 2.9 Strength of evidence

Type I   Strong evidence from at least one systematic review of multiple well-designed randomised controlled trials (RCTs)

Type II   Strong evidence from at least one properly designed randomised controlled trial of appropriate size

Type III Evidence from well-designed trials without randomi-
sation, single group pre–post, cohort, time-series or
matched case–control studies
Type IV Evidence from well-designed non-experimental studies
from more than one centre or research group
Type V Opinions of respected authorities, based on clinical
evidence, descriptive studies or reports of expert
committees

This hierarchy of evidence can be simplified into an ABC format.[6]

- A – at least one randomised controlled trial required as part of the
  body of literature of overall good quality and consistency addressing a
  specific recommendation.
- B – availability of well-conducted clinical studies required, but no
  randomised clinical trials on the topic of recommendation.
- C – evidence required that has been obtained from expert committee reports or opinions and/or clinical experiences of respected
  authorities; indicates absence of directly applicable clinical studies
  of good quality.

Other categories of evidence are listed in the compendium of the best
available evidence for effective healthcare – *Clinical Evidence* – which
is updated every six months. This categorisation of evidence is perhaps
more useful to the health professional in everyday work (*see* Box 2.10)[16]

Box 2.10

Beneficial	Interventions whose effectiveness has been shown by clear evidence from controlled trials
Likely to be beneficial	Interventions for which effectiveness is less well established than for those listed under 'beneficial'
Trade-off between benefits and harm	Interventions for which clinicians and patients should weigh up the beneficial and harmful effects according to individual circumstances and priorities
Unknown effectiveness	Interventions for which there are currently insufficient data, or data

	of inadequate quality (this includes interventions that are widely accepted as beneficial but which have never been formally tested in randomised control trials (RCTs), often because the latter would be regarded as unethical)
Unlikely to be beneficial	Interventions for which the lack of effectiveness is less well established than for those listed under 'likely to be ineffective or harmful'
Likely to be ineffective or harmful	Interventions whose ineffectiveness or harmfulness has been demonstrated by clear evidence

The Scottish Intercollegiate Guidelines Network (SIGN) has produced over 50 evidence-based guidelines. They base their recommendations on systematic reviews of the scientific literature. SIGN sees local ownership of the implementation of guidelines as crucial to success in changing practice. There are SIGN guidelines on *Obesity in Scotland: integrating prevention and weight management.*[6]

Accountability and performance

Health professionals may not always realise that they are accountable to others from outside their own professions, especially if they are of self-employed status, as are GPs, pharmacists and optometrists. However, in fact they are accountable to:

- the general public
- the profession – to maintain the standards of knowledge and skills of the profession as a whole
- the Government – and employer – who expect high standards of healthcare from the workforce.

Identify and rectify under-performance at an early stage by, for example:

- regular appraisals (at least annually) linked to clinical governance and personal development plans; appraisals should be supportive meetings, but need a mechanism for dealing with under-performance if it occurs

- detecting clinicians who have significant health problems, and referring them for help
- systematic audit that distinguishes individuals' performance from the overall performance of the practice team
- an open learning culture in which team members are discouraged from covering up colleagues' inadequacies, so that problems can be resolved at an early stage.

Clinicians may regard the performance assessment framework as a management tool that is not particularly relevant to their clinical practice. However, it does reinforce a clinical governance culture whereby good clinical and organisational management have a symbiotic relationship.

Box 2.11 The NHS performance assessment framework has six components

Examples of indicators that might be used to measure local performance include the following:[17]

- *health improvement*: incidence and prevalence of obesity-related diseases in a local population, such as those with type 2 diabetes
- *fair access*: access to a dietitian across the local area
- *efficiency*: cost per person of maintaining 1 kg of weight loss per year by type of service
- *effective delivery of appropriate care*: number and percentage of overweight and/or obese individuals with an associated comorbidity or relevant risk factor who have received advice/treatment according to an agreed protocol in a PCO or practice
- *user/carer experience*: length of time for which it is necessary to wait to see a dietitian
- *health outcomes*: percentage of the target population who achieve and/or maintain their recommended BMI level over a specific length of time.

Health promotion

There is a direct linear association between body mass index and coronary morbidity and mortality. The lower the BMI, the lower the risk a person has of heart disease and type 2 diabetes. Adults whose BMI lies in the upper realm of the 'normal' BMI range can decrease their risks of cardiovascular disease and diabetes by reducing their weight, as the research report in Box 2.12 shows.

Box 2.12

A prospective American study of 100 000 nurses aged 30 to 55 years found that the relative risk of coronary heart disease for women with a BMI of 25–28.9 was approximately twice that of women whose BMI was less than 21. The association of BMI with the risk of type 2 diabetes was even stronger. Women with a BMI of 23–23.9 had a 3.6-fold increase in risk compared with women with a BMI of less than 22.[18]

A rise in sedentary behaviour and a decline in physical activity are thought to explain much of the increasing trend towards overweight and obesity in the UK. Only a quarter of women and just over one-third of men were found to be engaged in regular, moderate physical activity in one recent national study.[8]

Good information will help people with coronary heart disease to make choices about their diet, smoking, physical activity and other health-related behaviour. Lifelong exercise and the avoidance of overweight and obesity seem to protect against the risk of stroke.[12]

It is well known that GPs' longer consultation times are linked with better quality of care.[19] Health promotion and opportunistic counselling about weight management are much more likely to occur if doctors are consulting at 10-minute intervals rather than shorter times.

Box 2.13 Effects of weight loss on respiratory function[20]

Weight loss reduces airways obstruction as well as peak expiratory flow variability in obese people who have asthma. The results of a study of 14 obese asthma patients who were studied before and after a very-low-calorie diet of eight weeks duration suggest that obese patients benefit from weight loss by 'improved pulmonary mechanics and a better control of airways obstruction'.

Another concern is preventing patients from losing so much weight as a result of social or internal pressures that they go to the opposite extreme of significant underweight (BMI $< 18.5\,\text{kg/m}^2$). They are then at risk of osteoporosis. Bone density will increase in response to weight gain.

Audit and evaluation

Audit will probably be the method you think of first for assessing how well you are doing and what it is you need to learn.

You might look at the extent to which you are adhering to practice protocols – for instance, whether you are giving consistent advice about weight and exercise to everyone at risk for cardiovascular disease and/or diabetes, or the extent to which you achieve health outcomes (*see* Box 2.11 for an example).

You could undertake a significant event audit in connection with a clinical problem arising, such as an obese adolescent developing type 2 diabetes. This would involve reviewing the opportunities that the practice team had had for giving opportunistic advice to the parents and the teenager about weight management throughout his or her childhood.

Core requirements

You cannot deliver clinical governance without well-trained and competent staff, the right skill mix of staff, and a safe and comfortable working environment.

The NHS Plan for England[21] describes the core requirements for the NHS which are part of a clinical governance culture in relation to the following:

- *partnership*: working together across the NHS to ensure the best possible care
- *performance*: acting to review and deliver higher standards of healthcare
- *the professions and wider workforce*: breaking down barriers between different disciplines (e.g. through multidisciplinary teamwork between GPs and nurses with pharmacists and other independent contractors)
- *patient care*: access, convenient services, and empowerment to take a full part in decision making about their own medical care and in planning and providing health services in general
- *prevention*: promoting healthy living across all sections of society and tackling variations in care.

Risk management

People may underestimate relative risks as applied to themselves and their own behaviour – for example, many smokers accept the relationship between smoking tobacco and disease, but do not believe that they personally are at risk. People usually have a reasonable idea of the *relative risks* of various activities and behaviours, although their personal estimates of the *magnitude* of those risks tend to be biased – small probabilities are often over-estimated and high probabilities are often under-estimated.[3]

Risk management in general practice mainly centres on assessing probabilities that potential or actual hazards will give rise to harm. Consider how bad the risk is, how likely the risk is, when the risk will occur if ever, and how certain you are of estimates about the risk. This applies just as much whether the risk is an environmental or organisational risk within the practice, or a clinical risk.

Box 2.14 Relative risk of different diseases in obese vs. non-obese individuals[8]

The risk for a non-obese individual is taken as 1 and the relative risk of an obese individual developing the disease is given in comparison for men and women.

Disease	*Relative risk*
Type 2 diabetes	
Women	12.7
Men	5.2
Hypertension	
Women	4.2
Men	2.6
Heart attack	
Women	3.2
Men	1.5
Colon cancer	
Women	2.7
Men	3.0
Angina	
Women	1.8
Men	1.8
Gall-bladder disease	
Women	1.8
Men	1.8
Ovarian cancer	
Women	1.7
Osteoarthritis	
Women	1.4
Men	1.9
Stroke	
Women	1.3
Men	1.3

Good practice means understanding and managing risk (both clinical and organisational aspects). Undertaking audit more systematically will reduce the risks of omission. Common areas of risk in providing healthcare services include:[3]

- out-of-date clinical practice
- lack of continuity of care
- poor communication
- mistakes in patient care
- patient complaints
- financial risk – insufficient resources
- reputation
- staff morale.

Communicating and managing risks on an individual basis with patients depends on finding ways to explain risks and elicit people's values and preferences. They can then make decisions themselves to take risks or choose between alternatives that involve different risks and benefits.

Having a system for gathering patients' comments or a good patient complaint system should reduce the risk of a recurrence of the event which originally triggered the complaint.

Reflection exercise

Exercise 3

Review and plan your management of obesity using the 14 components of clinical governance as a checklist. Think how you might integrate these components of clinical governance into your personal development plan or your practice personal and professional development plan. Examples are given for each component listed below. Complete this yourself from your own perspective.

- *Establishing a learning culture*: e.g. informal discussion about obesity guidelines between GPs, nurses and the community pharmacist.
- *Managing resources and services*: e.g. review the roles and responsibilities for the management of obesity by members of the practice team and attached staff.

- *Establishing a research and development culture*: e.g. share among the practice team findings in key research papers on best practice when preventing and managing obesity.
- *Reliable and accurate data*: e.g. keep electronic records (both individual and team) so that everyone uses the same Read codes (or SNOMED; *see* page 24) and enters data consistently. Any audit exercises can be repeated next year and the results compared.
- *Evidence-based practice and policy*: e.g. update an evidence-based protocol for managing obesity and ensure that the management plan is incorporated into other relevant protocols (e.g. for coronary heart disease and diabetes).
- *Confidentiality*: e.g. check that everyone is adhering to your agreed code of practice for giving results or advice at the reception desk.
- *Health gain*: e.g. target patients with osteoarthritis of the knee for particular efforts in reducing the weight of those with above or below normal BMI values.
- *Coherent team*: e.g. communicate to the rest of your practice team new systems for classifying obesity or other risk factors for hypertension or coronary heart disease.
- *Audit and evaluation*: e.g. undertake a significant event audit and act on the findings to improve the quality of the management of obesity.
- *Meaningful involvement of patients and the public*: e.g. listen to and act on the comments of those who are obese about the care and services that you are providing.
- *Health promotion*: e.g. obtain or write literature promoting physical activity through local walks.
- *Risk management*: e.g. establish systems and procedures to identify, analyse and control clinical risks such as those arising from poor repeat-prescribing practices.
- *Accountability and performance*: e.g. keep good records of those who are obese, to demonstrate the outcomes of your management programmes.
- *Core requirements*: e.g. agree roles and responsibilities in the practice team, such as inter-team referrals for lifestyle advice.

Now that you have completed this interactive reflection exercise, transfer the information to the empty template of the personal development plan on pages 141–151 if you are working on your own learning plan, or to the practice personal and professional development plan on pages 165–172 if you are working on a practice team learning plan. Don't forget to keep the evidence of your learning in your personal portfolio.

References

1 Lilley R (1999) *Making Sense of Clinical Governance.* Radcliffe Medical Press, Oxford.

2 Chambers R and Wakley G (2000) *Making Clinical Governance Work For You.* Radcliffe Medical Press, Oxford.

3 Mohanna K and Chambers R (2001) *Risk Matters in Healthcare: communicating, explaining and managing risk.* Radcliffe Medical Press, Oxford.

4 Wakley G, Chambers R and Field S (2000) *Continuing Professional Development: making it happen.* Radcliffe Medical Press, Oxford.

5 Hooper L, Summerbell C, Higgins J *et al.* (2001) Dietary fat intake and prevention of cardiovascular disease: systematic review. *BMJ.* **322**: 757–63.

6 Scottish Intercollegiate Guidelines Network (SIGN) (1996) *Obesity in Scotland: integrating prevention with weight management.* SIGN, Edinburgh.

7 Stevens V, Obarzanek E, Cook N *et al.* (2001) Long-term weight loss and changes in blood pressure: results of the trials of hypertension prevention. Phase II. *Ann Intern Med.* **134**: 1–11.

8 National Audit Office (2001) *Tackling Obesity in England.* National Audit Office, London.

9 Miller C, Ross N and Freeman M (1999) *Shared Learning and Clinical Teamwork: new directions in education and multiprofessional practice.* The English National Board for Nursing, Midwifery and Health Visiting, University of Brighton, Brighton.

10 Chambers R (2000) *Involving Patients and the Public. How to do it better.* Radcliffe Medical Press, Oxford.

11 Hofman A and Vandenbroucke JP (1992) Geoffrey Rose's big idea. Changing the population distribution of a risk factor is better than targeting people at high risk. *BMJ.* **305**: 1519–20.

12 Hunt R, Rayner M and Sharp I (eds) (2000) *Health Update. Coronary heart disease and stroke.* Health Development Agency, London.

13 Department of Health (1997) Report of the review of patient-identifiable information. In: *The Caldicott Committee Report.* Department of Health, London.

14 Donald P (2000) Promoting local ownership of guidelines. *Guidelines Pract.* **3**: 17.

15 Muir Gray JA (1997) *Evidence-Based Healthcare.* Churchill Livingstone, Edinburgh.

16 Barton S (ed.) (2001) *Clinical Evidence. Issue 5.* BMJ Publishing Group, London.

17 Davis AM, Giles A and Rona R (2000) *Tackling Obesity. A toolbox for local partnership action.* Faculty of Public Health Medicine, Royal College of Physicians, London.

18 Liu S and Manson JE (2001) What is the optimal weight for cardiovascular health? *BMJ.* **322**: 631–2.

19 Howie JG, Porter A, Heaney D and Hopton J (1991) Long to short consultation ratio: a proxy measure of quality of care. *Br J Gen Pract.* **41**: 48–54.

20 Hakala K, Stenius-Aarniala B and Sovijarvi A (2000) Effects of weight loss on peak flow variability, airways obstruction and lung volumes in obese patients with asthma. *Chest.* **118**: 1315–21.

21 Department of Health (2000) *The NHS Plan.* Department of Health, London.

CHAPTER 3

Managing child obesity and overweight in primary care

The prevalence of overweight and obesity among children in the UK has risen sharply since the 1980s. The rising trend of overweight and obesity in adolescence seems to persist into adulthood. However, not all obese adults were fat as children, although fat children have a high risk of progressing to become fat adults.[1]

Determining overweight and obesity in children is complicated because the ratio of weight/height gain fluctuates during normal growth. BMI normally rises steeply in infants, falls during pre-school years, and then increases again up to adulthood, especially around puberty. Some classifications specify values above the 80th centile as 'overweight', as this corresponds to a BMI of 25 at the age of 18 years in men and women. Others use the 85th centile to describe 'overweight', and the 95th or 98th centiles as the cut-off figures for 'obesity', in combination with skinfold measures at the triceps. You should be sure what measurement has been used when statistics are cited – or if you are interpreting measurements for your own child population.[2,3]

An adult BMI index should not be attributed to an adolescent until he or she reaches maturity.

There are helpful charts and measures for assessing BMI in children and comparing these values with age- and height-related charts.[4] Experts have warned practice teams about the inaccuracies that result from the use of inappropriately sited height gauges fixed over skirting boards or radiators.

Around 4% of both boys and girls aged 2–15 years in the UK are above the 98th centile according to BMI reference curves created for UK children.[1]

The numbers of overweight children increased between 1984 and 1994 in the UK, as is shown in Table 3.1. Rates of overweight and obesity between 1974 and 1984 showed little change.[5]

Table 3.1 Prevalence rates of childhood overweight and obesity in the UK[5]

Increase in the prevalence of:	1984	1994
Boys who are overweight	5.6%	9.0%
Girls who are overweight	9.3%	13.5%
Boys who are obese		1.7%
Girls who are obese		2.6%

Scottish children seem to be gaining weight for their height faster than
English children. One study in Tayside in Scotland found that 20% of
children and adolescents were overweight.[5,6]

Rates of overweight and obesity among pre-school children are
increasing, too. A study of infants and pre-school children (97% of
whom were of white European origin) found that there had been a
highly significant increase in the proportion who were overweight or
obese in this age group over the decade up to 1998. Around 24% were
overweight (> 85th centile) and 9% were obese (> 95th centile) in 1998,
representing increases of 60% and 70%, respectively. The authors
concluded that any community-based interventions designed to
reduce the frequency of overweight and obesity should be targeted at
this young age group, too.[3]

Childhood obesity is more common in deprived communities. Children from poorer households are more likely to have other adverse risk
factors as well, leading to greater morbidity and mortality in adult life.

Health consequences

There are health and social consequences for obese children and
adolescents. Effects on health include increased blood lipids, hypertension, glucose intolerance (type 2 diabetes accounts for about one-
third of all new cases of diabetes in children in America), hypertension
and an increase in liver enzymes. It is thought that more than 60% of
overweight children have at least one additional risk factor for cardiovascular disease, such as raised blood pressure, hyperlipidaemia or
hyperinsulinaemia. More than 20% of overweight children have two
risk factors.[7]

Another study[2] has found that the risk of colorectal cancer and gout
was increased in men who were obese as adolescents, and the risk of
arthritis was increased in women who were obese as adolescents.

Obese children have also been found to under-perform at school. Children of normal weight may ridicule the obese child, who then becomes socially isolated from his or her peers. Research has shown that obese children are consistently rated by peers as being less active, less attractive, less healthy, weak-willed, and having poor self-control with regard to dietary habits.[8] Overweight adolescent girls have lower levels of educational achievement, lower incomes, and are less likely to marry than normal-weight teenage girls.[1]

Table 3.2 Health consequences of childhood obesity (modified from Garrow and Summerbell[1])

Common consequences	Occasional consequences	Uncommon consequences
Faster growth	Hepatic steatosis	Orthopaedic complications
Psychosocial problems	Abnormal glucose metabolism	Sleep apnoea
Persistence into adulthood (for late-onset and severe obesity)	Persistence into adulthood (depending on age of onset and severity)	Polycystic ovary syndrome
		Pseudotumour cerebri
Dyslipidaemia		Cholelithiasis
Elevated blood pressure		Hypertension

Not only does obesity in childhood increase the risks of obesity in adulthood, but also obesity in adolescence damages adult health – it is directly associated with increased morbidity and mortality in adult life, independent of adult body weight.[1]

Prevention of obesity in children

Family therapy was found to be more effective in preventing the progression of obesity in 10 to 11-year-olds than conventional dietary and exercise treatments or no intervention, in one research study.[9]

The extent of the influence of the family environment is well demonstrated in Box 3.1.

Box 3.1 Relationship between use of television during meals and children's food consumption patterns[10]

The diet of children from families in which television viewing is a normal part of meal routines may include less fruit and vegetables and more pizzas, snack foods and fizzy high-calorie drinks than that of children from families where television viewing and eating are separate activities.

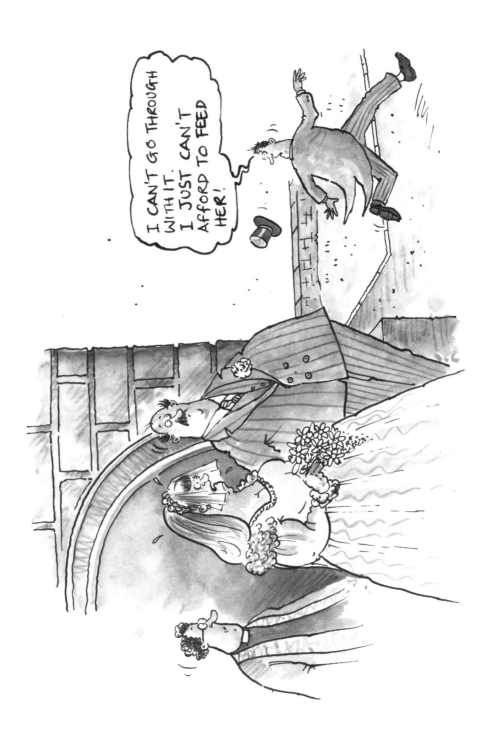

Nursery schools and schools should promote healthy eating and physical activity. National measures are needed to increase the availability of cheap and nutritious foods to families and children – through schools or by other means. It has been suggested that forbidding children to eat certain foods, such as those high in calories, may encourage them to overconsume these forbidden foods once they reach adolescence and adulthood and have uncontrolled access to them.[7] Thus children of food-controlling parents may find it more difficult to regulate their own food intake in a sensible way when they grow up.

Treatment of obesity in children

The most effective approach advocated by all authorities[1,7,9] is to:

- reduce sedentary behaviour and encourage all types of physical activity and play by reducing inactive time such as television viewing
- substitute fruit and low-energy drinks for sweets and high-energy drinks
- reduce the high fat content of the diet
- encourage the child to make sensible food choices.

Many studies have implicated sugary drinks as a cause of excess calorie intake – and advocated their substitution with artificially sweetened drinks.

Aim for a slowing of weight gain rather than weight loss, allowing the child to 'grow into' their current BMI if they are pre-pubertal.

It is not certain whether involving the parents in treatment programmes improves the outcome. Such involvement is probably more useful for children under eight years of age.[9] However, it makes sense to teach all parents about what constitutes a healthy diet and about the benefits of physical activity, as part of any approach to tackling child overweight and obesity, and to encourage them to act as healthy role models for their children. It may be counter-productive to involve the parents when advising an adolescent about losing excess weight. Encourage teenagers to take personal responsibility as far as possible, and follow the advice about behavioural therapies in Chapter 6.[2]

Behavioural modification, such as that employed when changing physical activity habits, works better with reinforcement – for example, by providing rewards for 'good' behaviour.[9]

Reflection exercise

Exercise 4

Were you previously aware of how common overweight and obesity in childhood are becoming? Had you noted the problem in your own practice population? You could find out more about this subject by reading some of the in-depth texts cited in the chapter.

Could you intervene more often (e.g. at the postnatal check, or as children present during routine consultations)? Could you work more closely with the health visitor and school nurse to reduce the prevalence of childhood overweight and obesity in your practice population? Consider convening an informal meeting in the practice for all those who are interested. Ask the practice manager to find out what records you have for BMI in children, and pool your records with those to which the health visitor and school nurse have access. Make an action plan to learn more about the problem of obesity in children and be pro-active in helping those identified as having a weight problem to slow their weight gain or reduce their weight as appropriate.

> Now that you have completed this interactive reflection exercise, transfer the information to the empty template of the personal development plan on pages 141–151 if you are working on your own learning plan, or to the practice personal and professional development plan on pages 165–172 if you are working on a practice team learning plan. Don't forget to keep the evidence of your learning in your personal portfolio.

References

1 Garrow J and Summerbell C (2002) Obesity. In: *Health Care Needs Assessment*. Third Series. Radcliffe Medical Press, Oxford.

2 Garrow J (chair) (1999) *Obesity. Report of the British Nutrition Foundation Task Force*. Blackwell Science, Oxford.

3 Bundred P, Kitchiner D and Buchan I (2000) Prevalence of overweight and obese children between 1989 and 1998: population-based series of cross-sectional studies. *BMJ*. **320**: 326–8.

4 Fry T (2000) Beating childhood obesity. *J Assoc Prim Care Groups Trusts*. **1**: 103–9.

5 Chinn S and Rona RJ (1994) Trends in weight for height and triceps skinfold thickness for English and Scottish children, 1972–1982 and 1982–1990. *Paediatr Perinat Epidemiol.* **8**: 90–106.

6 Scottish Intercollegiate Guidelines Network (SIGN) (1996) *Obesity in Scotland: integrating prevention with weight management.* SIGN, Edinburgh.

7 Dietz W (2001) The obesity epidemic in young children. *BMJ.* **322**: 313–14.

8 National Audit Office (2001) *Tackling Obesity in England.* National Audit Office, London.

9 NHS Centre for Reviews and Dissemination (1997) The prevention and treatment of obesity. *Effective Health Care Bull.* **3**: 1–12.

10 Coon K, Goldberg J, Rogers B *et al.* (2001) Relationships between use of television during meals and children's food consumption patterns. *Paediatrics.* **107**: 1–9.

CHAPTER 4

Managing adult overweight and obesity in primary care

Peter Stott

Healthcare professionals should take every opportunity to educate their patients, their families and society more generally with regard to the problems which may arise from being overweight or obese.

Management of obesity in adults begins with educating children at home and at school in order to prevent weight problems from arising. More attention should be paid to education about what constitutes a healthy diet, and providing safe walking routes to school and adequate resources to fund physical and recreational activities. For adults, the workplace can promote reasonable levels of physical activity, ensure opportunities for healthy low fat food choices and urge healthier lifestyles. The media could do more to promote sensible approaches to weight loss, and the food industry should share responsibility for making sensible and economic food choices available.

Managing within available resources

It is impractical and inappropriate for GP practices to take on the full burden of tackling obesity. The problem is not one of health alone. The responsibility for countering obesity crosses many government departments, and the solution will involve all of these working together. Transport policy, food policy, product labelling, agriculture, public broadcasting, schools, higher education, sport and entertainment all play a part. National and local government should work together in an integrated fashion.[1]

Liaison with other agencies is important. The minimisation of morbidity arising from overweight and obesity will require an integrated approach involving not only primary and secondary care, but also social services, private agencies and the media.

Nevertheless, because of our ongoing relationship with individuals and families, primary care team members have a key role in influencing change. Key priorities can be identified, even given the resource constraints within which we work. Many of the individuals at highest risk will already be attending practice clinics for diabetes, hyperlipidaemia or hypertension. Weight-management protocols can be grafted on to these clinics with minimal disruption and within the existing resources.

Government and local strategies

The National Service Framework for Coronary Heart Disease for England[2] advises that weight management and appropriate dietary advice underpins good preventive cardiovascular care. The Framework states that:

> General practitioners and primary healthcare teams should identify all people at significant risk of cardiovascular disease but who have not developed symptoms, and offer them appropriate advice and treatment.
>
> By April 2001, HAs, LAs, PCGs/PCTs and NHS trusts will have agreed and be contributing to the delivery of the local programme of effective policies on:
>
> - reducing smoking
> - promoting healthy eating
> - increasing physical activity
> - reducing overweight and obesity.
>
> By April 2002, HAs, LAs, PCGs/PCTs and NHS trusts (in England) will have quantitative data no more than 12 months old about implementation of these policies.

Achieving these targets without additional resources will be a major challenge for primary care organisations.

The large majority of health authorities in England have identified obesity as a public health priority in their health improvement

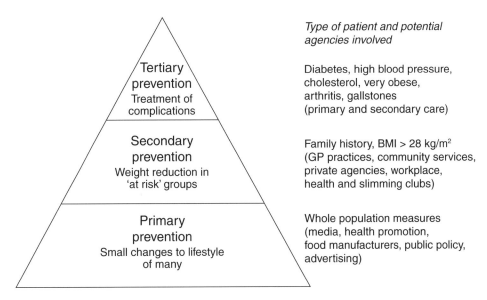

Figure 4.1: The iceberg of obesity.

programmes, but only a quarter had actually taken action to address it according to a recent report.[1]

The concept of the iceberg of risk provides a model which enables health professionals to understand the concept of risk (*see* Figure 4.1). It is widely used to illustrate how the three levels of interventions (primary, secondary and tertiary prevention) can influence the natural history of a disease and help to prioritise our efforts.

Primary prevention of obesity and overweight

Primary prevention works best when small changes are made to the lifestyles of many individuals. It may be mediated by television, radio and the press, health promotion activities, role models and peer pressure. These types of activities, although informed by clinicians, are largely the concern of public health policy.

Primary prevention of obesity and overweight can be undertaken in a range of situations and in a variety of ways. Those who are involved in the media and the making of public policy decisions should continue to keep the issue in public view as a 'hot' topic. Exposing people to healthy images with regard to physical form, fitness, diet and behaviour will

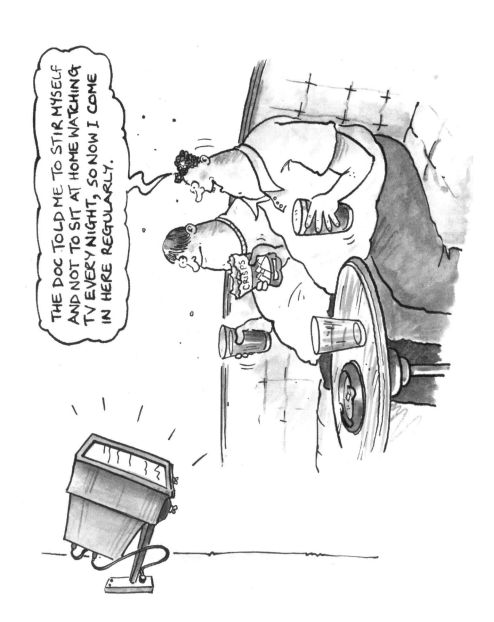

discourage obesity-provoking lifestyles. At first sight, many of the primary modes of prevention may seem tangential. For example, policies which encourage walking to work or school, public transport and cycling, and which discourage the ready use of cars, should all have a positive effect. Schoolchildren can have a particularly important influence on the eating and exercising behaviour of their parents.

Other ideas for prevention include the GP and nurse giving advice about weight management to those who are at risk of weight gain – for example, when a patient is obese or has type 2 diabetes, or is being prescribed drugs such as steroid therapy or contraceptive pills, or has become temporarily or permanently immobile.

Secondary prevention of obesity and overweight

Secondary prevention is targeted at those who are specifically at risk of a problem, and offers strategies which will reduce that risk. Secondary prevention in obesity management should involve seeking out those who are already very overweight (e.g. with a BMI of > 28) or obese, and offering help before complications develop. Since 95% of the practice population is seen every five years, such a task could be performed on an opportunistic basis. The average general practitioner with 1800 patients is likely to have 250 or more adult patients who are obese. It is probably unrealistic to expect practice teams to manage all of the obese patients themselves without extra funding. Although selected patients might be managed in the practice, the majority will probably be best directed to existing local services such as private slimming clubs and health promotion clinics.

Tertiary prevention of obesity

Tertiary prevention involves identifying individuals who have already developed a medical problem as a result of their condition, and managing them effectively in order to reduce the long-term risks due to progression of the disease. Hospital clinicians have little opportunity to undertake anything other than tertiary prevention.

Tertiary prevention should involve identifying obese individuals who have already developed complications and working with them to reduce the long-term consequences of their excessive weight. If practice teams start with weight management of their practice population at this level, where they know that the risk is high, they can extend their efforts into secondary prevention as data emerges and they become more clinically confident and adequate funds are allocated. This is the same approach that primary care teams have taken to managing hypertension, hyperlipidaemia and osteoporosis – first targeting those at most obvious risk, and then moving on to help those patients with lower risks.

There are three key groups who are most at risk of developing complications from overweight and obesity:

1 patients with a BMI of >28 who are already suffering from the secondary effects of obesity (e.g. type 2 diabetes, cardiovascular disease, hypercholesterolaemia, arthritis or hypertension)
2 patients who are obese (BMI $\geqslant 30$)
3 patients with higher levels of overweight (BMI 28–30) with a family history of obesity-related disease or who, having lost weight, are having difficulty in maintaining their weight.

Patients who are morbidly obese (BMI $\geqslant 40 \, \text{kg/m}^2$) are probably best managed in a specialist clinic (e.g. a diabetic clinic) where appropriate resources, such as access to a dietitian, are available.

Most of the patients at risk from their obesity may be identified opportunistically. If you wish to be more pro-active, run a computerised audit and reconcile records of BMI values with the relevant diagnosis or prescribed drugs.

Box 4.1

Primary care organisations could establish primary care weight control clinics as intermediate referral centres that provide access to community dietetics and specialist obesity services, with psychological and psychiatric services also available if appropriate.

Guidelines for the management of overweight and obesity

Three sets of obesity guidelines for overweight and obesity have been published in the UK:

1 *Integrating Prevention and Weight Management: The Scottish Intercollegiate Guidelines Network (SIGN) (1996)*[3]
2 *The Clinical Management of Overweight and Obese patients. The Royal College of Physicians (1998)*[4]
3 *The National Obesity Forum Guidelines, 2000*[5] (*see* Appendix 2).

These guidelines differ only in minor points. All of them emphasise the following four components that constitute the effective management of obesity:

• diet
• behavioural change
• increased physical activity
• drug treatment.

The individual who is overweight or obese must be motivated to change before any of these guidelines can be put into action. General practitioners and practice nurses will be well skilled in identifying patients who are ready and sufficiently motivated to make changes to their lifestyle. It is essential to choose an appropriate moment, just as when trying to help smokers, alcoholics and drug addicts to change their destructive habits. Individuals should have moved past the stage of contemplation and be well into the stage of taking action for themselves before practice resources are invested.

Figure 6.1 illustrates the different stages in the cycle of change (*see* Chapter 6). Nothing is so demotivating to a health professional as working very hard with an individual for several weeks, only to realise that the patient has not been taking the process seriously. Realistic targets should be set in the early days so as not to demotivate the patient or allow them an escape route ('I knew I couldn't do it'). Many of these people will have tried many times in the past to reduce their excess weight, and may have become easily demotivated. Professional advisers can often change this pattern.

Box 4.2

Be realistic about possible weight loss. Suggested targets for an obese person include the following:

• weight loss of 2.5 kg in the first four weeks
• 5% of body weight lost in three months
• 10% of body weight lost by one year.

A 10% loss of body weight over the course of one year is a realistic target for most people. This level of weight reduction has been shown to be associated with a number of health benefits, particularly if diabetes, hypertension or hyperlipidaemia are present.[2,6-11]

Box 4.3 Benefits of 10% loss of body weight in an obese person[3,6]

Mortality:
> 20% decrease in premature mortality
> 30% decrease in diabetes-related deaths.

Blood pressure:
10 mmHg decrease in systolic blood pressure
20 mmHg decrease in diastolic blood pressure.

Diabetes:
50% decrease in fasting glucose levels.

Lipids:
30% decrease in triglycerides
10% decrease in total cholesterol
15% decrease in LDL cholesterol
8% increase in HDL cholesterol.

Discuss and resolve any possible mismatch of agendas between the person who is overweight or obese and the health professional. Patients often regard weight management as the route to becoming a sylph (at the very least eligible for page 3 of a tabloid newspaper!). Health professionals are more concerned that the patient loses 10% of their body weight in order to become more healthy.

Diet

Formal calorie-counting diets may be useful for getting someone who is obese or overweight started on a weight-loss programme, but strict diets are difficult to sustain in the longer term. Most people like variety in their diet and they enjoy 'treats'. One of the most important aims of any programme is to help patients to recognise 'danger foods' (particularly those high in fat), and to help them to increase their own control over eating. In practice, a 600-calorie-deficient diet is normally effective.

Calorie counting and fat avoidance can be encouraged by asking the patient to keep a food diary, which can also provide insight when weight loss is not proceeding as planned.

It is common for obese and overweight individuals to underestimate their food intake by about one-third – perhaps because of genuine forgetfulness, or self-deception due to a lack of understanding of food composition, particularly with regard to hidden fat. In particular, the eating of snacks tends to be under-reported.

Food is an important part of social life. The diet should not be so defined as to prevent the patient enjoying normal social intercourse, or so strict as to preclude 'treats'. 'Negative dieting' is often counter-productive in the long term. The approach that should be taken should emphasise new food opportunities, new methods of food preparation, and the integration of 'treats' into the overall food plan.

Many patients will have stories of very-low-calorie or quirky diets which have helped them to lose vast amounts of weight rapidly in the past. Sadly, most of these patients will have relapsed subsequently. This emphasises one of the key messages – that a weight-control programme is not just a 'one-off' diet to give someone a rapid period of weight loss, but rather it is a process of re-education which will affect their whole lifestyle. It is relatively easy to lose weight over a short period, but much more difficult to maintain that weight loss over the longer term. Only improved insight, changed dietary habits, behavioural change and exercise will sustain optimal weight.

Box 4.4

The long-term aim is to give people control over what they eat, and not to let food control them.

More information about dietary approaches can be found in Chapter 5.

Physical activity

The Health Education Authority recommends that 'adults should try to build up gradually to take half an hour of moderate-intensity physical activity on five or more days of the week. Activities like brisk walking, cycling, swimming, dancing and gardening are good options'.[12]

One of the key insights which health professionals can give to patients involves forging a link between the calorific value of the food a person eats and the exercise which is necessary to burn off those calories. This is particularly useful in cases where the patient is prone to 'snacking'. Box 4.5 illustrates some typical activities together with their calorie and food equivalents. Most people find these comparisons surprising, and gasp with astonishment. Armed with concepts such as this, they will rapidly learn to recognise that if they eat something extra then it must be balanced with an equivalent extra energy output – otherwise they must expect an increase in body weight.

Box 4.5 Examples of exercise types and the calorie and food equivalents

Activity
   Energy expended per hour in kilocalories
   Food equivalent expended per hour

Driving a car
   80 kcal
   Slice of bread

Standing relaxed
   100 kcal
   Glass of white wine

Standing doing light work
   180 kcal
   Bag of crisps

Walking 5 km in an hour
   260 kcal
   1½ pints of beer

Walking 7 km in an hour
   420 kcal
   2½ oz peanuts

Running 9 km in an hour
   600 kcal
   Two chocolate bars

Cross-country skiing (competitive)
   1440 kcal
   Roast dinner with sponge pudding

The challenge to healthcare professionals is to drive these obvious healthcare messages home and to trigger action. Activities that are recommended must be realistic for the individual concerned and appropriate to any other problems they might have. There is little point in recommending a two mile walk to someone with severe airways disease, but they may be able to manage to climb their stairs once an hour or take a gentle walk to the shops. Activities which fit into the individual's lifestyle and which are easily put into action are the ones that are most likely to succeed in the long term.

For fitter individuals, suggest short 'triggers' such as climbing stairs, running for a bus or walking fast. Help patients to recognise that their longer periods of activity are beginning to pay dividends and that they are gradually becoming able to take on more, and to move faster and more easily.

Specific recommendations for physical activity for people who are obese (adapted from Fox[13])

1   Build up slowly towards 30 minutes of moderate-intensity activity a day. The 30 minutes can be accumulated throughout the day in 10 to 15-minute bouts. Moderate intensity means breathing slightly harder than normal, but still within the 'comfort zone' whereby the activity can be done whilst talking at the same time.
2   To achieve optimal weight loss, consider extending some sessions to 45 minutes or longer, as this will encourage the use of fat as an energy source.
3   Increase the amount of daily routine activity, such as gardening, shopping, housework, walking, etc.
4   Decrease the amount of time spent in sedentary activities, and try not to sit down for more than 30 minutes at a time.
5   The most effective activities for achieving weight loss are those that involve large muscle groups, which are aerobic in nature, such as walking, swimming or cycling.
6   Consider weight-bearing exercises such as walking and climbing stairs, as these help to conserve muscle mass and maintain strength and resting metabolic rate.
7   Find physical activities which are enjoyable.

More information about the benefits of physical activity and effective interventions can be found in Chapter 6.

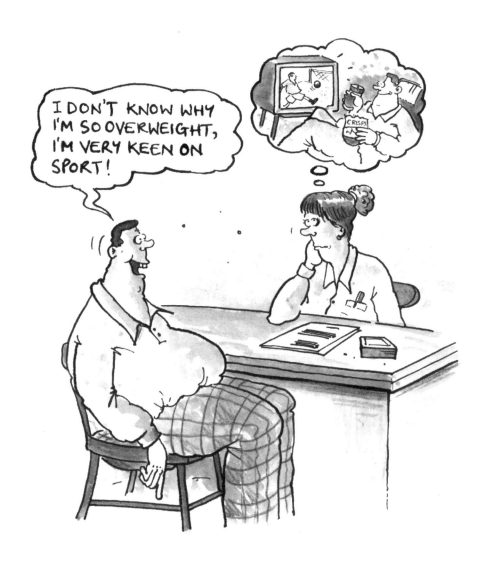

Behavioural change

The concept of human beings as hunter-gatherers has been replaced in the western world by humans as 'grazing animals', snacking their way from a breakfast of yoghurt and toast, through coffee and Danish pastries, the occasional chocolate bar, nuts and buns, to burger and fries followed by a chocolate pastry, a pizza dinner and a cereal snack before bedtime – all washed down with copious cappucinos, soft drinks and alcohol. Such fast and accessible food is also all too often fatty food, heavy in calories. It is specifically manufactured in this way so that it remains fresh for long periods during which it can be transported to the point of sale.

Some individuals behave in more obesity-provoking ways than others. Some snack on chocolate or crisps when they are stressed, while others socialise by means of food or alcohol. Teenagers prove their peer-group status with specific brands of fizzy drinks. Mothers put off eating properly until their partner returns home, but assuage their hunger with crisps. They finish off their children's dinners because 'they simply can't bear to see them leave food on their plate'. Some occupations put individuals more at risk than others. It is difficult for men working in the transport industries to find healthy food when they are on the move, and they tend to rely instead on fast but fatty food prepared in wayside cabins. Some people find that travelling home by public transport takes them temptingly close to coffee and pastry stalls. Other workers return home to an empty house where they snack on nuts and alcohol until their dinner is ready, perhaps an hour later.

It is as if the twenty-first century lifestyle has been specifically designed to provoke obesity and overweight. Food outlets tempt us throughout the day, wherever we are, and it is now rare to find a family with defined mealtimes taking meals together. Eating together is not only a social activity which strengthens family bonds, but it also focuses meals on specific time points in the day and allows hunger to develop before the next food intake. However, it is now common for individuals to eat every hour or so, with the result that their stomachs are never empty – no wonder their physiology is confused.

Obese and overweight individuals need to develop insight into behaviours such as these which they will need to change if they are to tackle their weight problem effectively. They must learn to feel and accept hunger again. It can be a time-consuming process, and the availability of a dietitian or food counsellor may be helpful.

There are four main aims of behavioural counselling:

- to increase awareness of attitudes to body weight, food and activity
- to identify inappropriate behaviours that cause and sustain obesity (e.g. snacking during periods of stress, finishing off children's meals)
- to present options for change based on a low-fat eating plan and increased physical activity
- to help patients to gain control and develop self-esteem.

More information about behavioural therapy can be found in Chapter 6.

Drug therapy

A number of alternatives are available to patients:

- agents which reduce fat absorption – for example, orlistat (Xenical) decreases fat absorption by inhibiting the enzyme lipase
- centrally acting appetite suppressants, although many (e.g. phentermine) have been discontinued because of associated problems such as pulmonary hypertension and heart-valve abnormalities; sibutramine is a serotonin and noradrenaline re-uptake inhibitor
- oat-based fat substitutes such as olestra
- methylcellulose – a bulk-forming agent which is claimed to reduce food intake by inducing satiety, although there is no evidence from randomised controlled trials that it is effective.

Drug treatment should always be combined with diet and behaviour management, and patients selected for drug treatment should have demonstrated that they are motivated by achieving a weight loss of at least 2.5 kg on diet alone in the first four weeks. More details on drug treatment can be found in Chapter 7.

Practice-based weight-control clinics

Structured multidisciplinary care can be provided in primary care through nurse-led clinics. Nurses are well placed to offer advice and support to help overweight or obese patients to adhere to their weight management programmes. The protocol in Box 4.6 gives an example of how an experienced nurse in one general practice is successfully managing their obese patients with support from the general practitioners.

The reflection exercises at the end of this chapter will help you to identify your learning needs and follow a detailed plan to set up a weight-management programme and compose a practice protocol for a nurse-led obesity clinic.

Box 4.6

In one practice that runs a weight-management clinic for patients who are obese, about one-third of patients achieve a 10% weight loss within the year, one-third lose 5–10%, and one-third lose no weight at all. This gives the practice weight loss programme a number needed to treat (NNT) of 3, which is rather better than that achieved with histamine 2 antagonists for duodenal ulcer.

Patients are managed according to the principles described in published guidelines,[3,4] incorporating dietary change, exercise, behaviour change, and drugs where appropriate. One of the GPs, a trained practice nurse and a dietitian work together in an integrated manner in a formal clinic setting. They offer opportunistic appointments and education sessions in the evening. An exercise programme is also available for suitable patients. Following the guidelines in this practice results in about one-third of patients receiving drug therapy.

Dr Peter Stott, Tadworth, Surrey

Two algorithms follow (*see* Figures 4.2 and 4.3). You could choose either one and adapt it to fit in with your approach to weight management and its ease of use for your practice team.

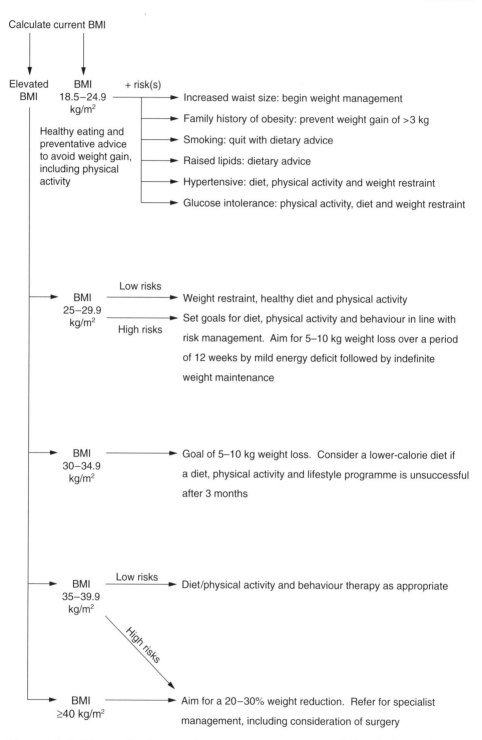

Figure 4.2: Example 1: weight management in adults (adapted from SIGN[3]).

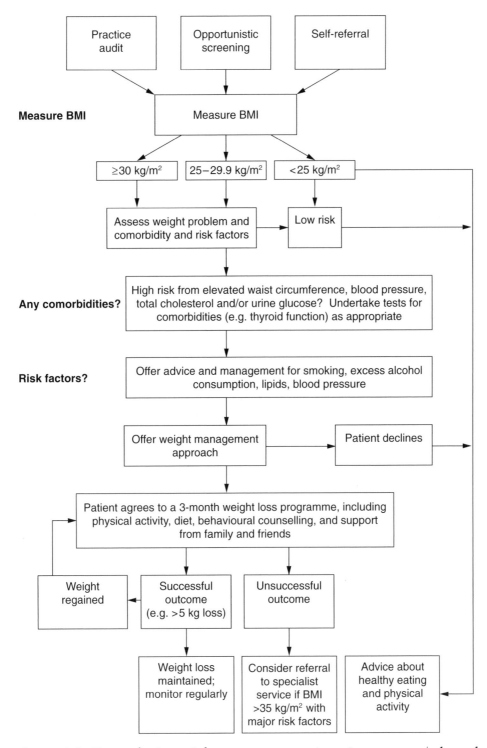

Figure 4.3: Example 2: weight management in primary care (adapted from SIGN[3]).

Reflection exercises

Exercise 5

Do you have a practice protocol for a weight-management programme?
Do all clinicians give consistent messages about weight reduction and
control? If not, you might want to follow the guidance below in order to
set up your own programme.

You could use this ten-step programme to set up a weight-management
programme in primary care.

1 Be realistic about what you can achieve, and don't expect too
   much. Trials have shown that around 15% of obese patients can
   lose 10% or more of their body weight in a year using non-
   pharmacological approaches.
2 Devise a practice strategy for tackling obesity. There should be four
   main components to your strategy:
   • dietary control (a low-fat, calorie-restricted diet, usually a
     reduction of around 600 kcal per day)
   • behavioural change (in order to avoid trigger situations and
     encourage such avoidance behaviours)
   • increased physical activity (regular sustained aerobic activity is
     sufficient)
   • drug treatment.
3 Start with those who are most at risk. Primary care resources are
   limited and should be directed at those who are most likely to
   benefit. Start with patients at the tip of the risk pyramid (*see*
   page 51).
4 Catch patients when they are motivated. The more highly motivated the patient is, the more likely he or she is to succeed in losing
   weight. Too many patients enter weight-loss programmes because
   family, friends and professional advisers persuade them to do so. A
   sense of personal motivation is essential. The time should be right
   – if there is too much going on in the patient's life, they may
   become distracted from the weight-reduction programme.
5 Involve as many other agencies as you can. Liaise with other
   agencies (e.g. the dietetic service, local sports facilities and gyms,
   private slimming organisations and occupational health services).
   This is particularly useful for overweight patients who do not
   fall into the most at-risk categories, and whom it would not be
   cost-effective for the practice to manage.

6 Involve your local dietitian. Dietary control is essential in the management of obesity. Modern diets tend to be relatively low in carbohydrates and high in fat, so emphasise calorie counting and avoiding fatty foods. The availability of a dietitian could be a marker of the quality of a primary care organisation.

7 Use your dietitian, practice nurse or health visitor to advise patients about behavioural changes. Counselling about potential behavioural change takes up a considerable amount of time. Initial counselling and follow-up sessions often take between 15 and 30 minutes. Behavioural counselling may be better suited to the skills of a nurse or dietitian than to those of a doctor. However, whoever takes on this role should be specially trained to look further than the clinical needs of the patient, to his or her day-to-day life.

8 Involve local gyms and fitness centres. Physical activity increases energy output, enhances fat loss and prevents weight gain. It also serves to reduce risk factors and increase personal motivation, confidence and self-esteem.

   Formal attendance at a gym or fitness centre is not absolutely necessary, and can sometimes be deleterious if it results in an increased appetite. Regular daily activity, such as walking the children to school, using public transport rather than a car, climbing stairs rather than using the lift, or joining a dance club, is adequate provided that it takes place often enough.

   Encourage patients to exercise aerobically to the limits of their fitness and to the point where conversation is just starting to become difficult.

9 Use drug therapy according to rigid criteria. Such therapy is an adjunct to diet, exercise and behavioural change – it is not a substitute, and should only be used in selected patients under strict medical guidance (*see* Chapter 7 for more details).

10 Persuade your primary care organisation to devote resources to the management of obesity.

   Share your practice expertise in managing obesity with others who wish to learn how you achieved your success. Primary care organisations are likely to devote more resources to the management of obesity, since it is a target within the National Service Framework for Coronary Heart Disease for England.[2] Other countries may follow suit.

Exercise 6

Are all members of the practice team (including the receptionists and other non-clinical staff) familiar with the standard approaches in your practice protocol for managing overweight and obesity? If not, review your clinic protocol at a practice team meeting. Ensure that everyone knows what their roles and responsibilities are. You might want to compare your practice protocol for obesity management with the example of a nurse-led clinic given below. If you do not run such a chronic disease clinic, why not set one up?

Protocol for a nurse-led, obesity-management programme

(Tadworth Medical Centre, courtesy of Sister Francina Hyatt)

Aim of the clinic: to help patients to achieve weight loss which will benefit their overall health, using lifestyle and behavioural approaches, and in some cases drug therapy.

Target weight loss: 10% of total body weight in a year.

Referral criteria: patients with comorbidities (e.g. diabetes, hypertension, hyperlipidaemia), whose BMI is greater than 28 kg/m^2, referred from other clinics or via their GP. Patients will be expected to be highly motivated to lose weight, and to have scored positively on the motivational assessment questionnaire.

Nurse's responsibility

First appointment (30 minutes)

1 Initial assessment:
   - discuss the patient's reasons for wanting to lose weight
   - explain the aim of the clinic and discuss the commitment required by the patient
   - assess obesity-related factors (e.g. family history, alcohol intake, high-fat diet) and record them on computer
   - discuss the benefits of weight loss.
2 Record baseline investigations:
   - current weight
   - waist circumference
   - blood pressure and pulse rate
   - urinalysis
   - cholesterol (if not previously estimated)

- HbA$_{1c}$ where type 2 diabetes has been previously diagnosed
- current medications.
3 Dietary assessment:
   - calculate basal metabolic index using standard equation or software
   - determine target weight and daily calorific intake per day, and enter them in the patient's weight-management diary
   - demonstrate use of the energy food portion table and food portion size sheets.
4 Behaviour:
   - assess the patient's obesity-related behaviours (e.g. place of eating, temptation to overeat, meal frequency, alcohol intake, etc.), and counsel them appropriately.
5 Physical activity:
   - emphasise the importance of increasing physical activity, and identify appropriate activities which can be performed for 30 minutes each day.
6 Further information:
   - provide an obesity information pack, and offer telephone support if required
   - tell the patient about the evening group meetings
   - offer a date for review in one month's time.

Follow-up appointment (15 minutes)

1 General:
   - initiate a general discussion about the changed eating patterns and how they have affected the patient's life
   - discuss the diary entries and any problems encountered.
2 Investigations:
   - weight and waist circumference
   - blood pressure, HbA$_{1c}$ for diabetes, and cholesterol after three months if appropriate.
3 Diet:
   - refer the patient to a dietitian for motivational counselling and dietetic advice if it is felt that further support would be helpful.
4 Exercise:
   - discuss the patient's activity level
   - prepare a specific plan where necessary (using computer program).
5 Drug therapy:
   - if at least 2.5 kg of weight loss has not been achieved after one month on the diet, consider whether drug treatment would be

helpful. Refer the patient to the doctor for further discussion of this step
- if the patient is already on drug treatment, then weigh them monthly to confirm a continued weight loss. Review the patient for any possible adverse drug reactions or interactions with other therapies, and arrange a further prescription where necessary. If weight loss is not maintained, then refer the patient back to the doctor for further advice on stopping therapy.

6 General:
- encourage self-monitoring of weight, food and activity by recording entries in the patient diary
- praise the patient for the progress they have made so far.

Doctor's responsibility

This is as follows:

- to be a source of advice and support to the nurse and the patients involved in the clinic
- to assess the suitability of patients referred by the nurse for drug therapy, and to prescribe any drug as appropriate
- to assist in organising group educational meetings.

Signatures:

I have read and understood this protocol. I have been trained in the relevant procedures and feel confident to carry out the tasks involved.

Signed:

. . . .

Nurse: Date: Doctor: Date:

Exercise 7

Undertake an audit of 20 patients, each of whom has received lifestyle advice about their raised body mass index. If you cannot identify such patients from the practice computer records, then select the cases for audit as consecutive patients present to a GP or practice nurse. Look back at their records to see when they were given lifestyle advice, by whom, and what the outcome has been. Does one member of staff have better success rates than the others? If so, can others learn more about motivating patients to change? Has everyone adhered to the practice protocol?

Now that you have completed these interactive reflection exercises, transfer the information to the empty template of the personal development plan on pages 141–151 if you are working on your own learning plan, or to the practice personal and professional development plan on pages 165–172 if you are working on a practice team learning plan. Don't forget to keep the evidence of your learning in your personal portfolio.

References

1 National Audit Office (2001) *Tackling Obesity in England*. National Audit Office, London.

2 Department of Health (2000) *National Service Framework for Coronary Heart Disease*. Department of Health, London.

3 Scottish Intercollegiate Guidelines Network (SIGN) (1996) *Obesity in Scotland: integrating prevention with weight management*. SIGN, Edinburgh.

4 Royal College of Physicians of London (1998) *Clinical Management of Overweight and Obese Patients, With Particular Reference to the Use of Drugs*. Royal College of Physicians of London, London.

5 National Obesity Forum (2000) *NOF Guidelines for the Management of Obesity in Adults*. National Obesity Forum, Nottingham.

6 Maryon Davis A, Giles A and Rona R (2000) *Tackling Obesity: a toolbox for local partnership action*. Faculty of Public Health, Royal Colleges of Physicians of the UK, London.

7 Manson JE, Willett WC, Stampfer MJ *et al.* (1995) Body weight and mortality among women. *NEJM*. **333**: 677–85.

8 Goldstein DJ (1992) Beneficial health effects of modest weight loss. *Int J Obesity.* **16**: 397–415.

9 Wing RR, Koeske R, Epstein LH *et al.* (1987) Long-term effects of modest weight loss in type II diabetic patients. *Arch Intern Med.* **147**: 1749–53.

10 Lean MEJ, Powrie JK, Anderson AS *et al.* (1990) Obesity, weight loss and prognosis in type 2 diabetes. *Diabet Med.* **7**: 228–33.

11 Dattilo AM and Kris-Etherton PM (1992) Effects of weight reduction on blood lipids and lipoproteins: a meta-analysis. *Am J Clin Nutr.* **56**: 320–28.

12 Health Education Authority (1998) *Managing Weight. A workbook for health and other professionals.* Health Education Authority, London.

13 Fox K (1999) Treatment of obesity. III. Physical activity and exercise. In: *Obesity. Report of the British Nutrition Foundation Task Force.* Blackwell Science, Oxford.

CHAPTER 5

Different dietary approaches

The aim of weight management should be to educate the person who is overweight or obese about the advantages to their health of losing weight, to help them to understand the reasons for their state, and to agree modest treatment goals and longer-term strategies for losing weight and sustaining that weight loss.

A mildly hypocaloric diet and exercise and behaviour modification programmes are the recommended approach.[1-3] The reasons for setting a target such as a 10% body weight loss over a year have been given in previous chapters. Losing 5 kg of fat requires a deficit of 35 000 kilo-calories (kcal). Losing this in two weeks means eating 2500 less kilo-calories per day, whilst losing it in four weeks means eating 1250 less kilocalories a day – or undertaking the equivalent amount of exercise. A more realistic target for someone who is obese might be to lose 10 kg over 6 to 12 months, which would require a deficit of 500–600 or 250–300 kilocalories, respectively, per day.[4,5]

Box 5.1

The combination of a calorie-restricted diet and exercise appears to be more beneficial for weight loss than a restricted diet alone, but light exercise (e.g. callisthenics and stretching) may be just as effective as moderate aerobic exercise (e.g. walking).[6]

The Scottish Intercollegiate Guidelines Network (SIGN) recommends a family approach to dietary change so that all members of the person's household are involved too.[1] This has the added advantages of setting a good role model for children if an overweight or obese parent is reducing their excessive weight and establishing a healthy diet as a norm.

A healthy diet

A healthy diet is one in which the various food groups are well balanced. The Committee on Medical Aspects of Food Policy (COMA) recommends a reduction in fat, particularly saturated fat, a reduction in salt and an increase in carbohydrate, especially that which is rich in fibre, for the UK population as a whole.[7] The Committee has recommended that the general population should increase their consumption of fruit, vegetables, bread and potatoes by 50% of current levels. Carbohydrates would then supply 50% of dietary energy and be a substitute for the reduced intake of fat. The current proportion of energy derived from fat is 38% of an average person's diet.

Fruit and vegetables are rich sources of potassium, which is associated with lower blood pressure levels and a lower risk of stroke.[7] The risk of cancer is also minimised by dietary changes. Up to 80% of bowel and breast cancer is thought to be preventable by dietary modification. In general, fruit and vegetables have a protective effect, whereas red and processed meats increase the risk of developing cancer. Current recommendations are to eat at least five portions of fruit and vegetables per day.[8]

Tips for a 'less fat diet' (adapted from the Food Standards Agency[9])

Fat contains twice as many calories as starch or protein of the same weight.

- Beware of invisible fats such as those found in foods like biscuits, cakes, chocolate, pastry and savoury snacks. Read the labels.
- Trim fat from meat and poultry.
- Opt for lower-fat milk, dairy products and spreads.
- Choose to bake or grill food rather than frying it (e.g. use oven chips instead of fried potatoes).
- Fill up on bread, cereals, potatoes, fruit and vegetables.
- Choose low-fat snacks to suit your taste.

Examples of well-known diets

While consulting health professionals, patients often talk about the particular diet they are trying out. Below is a brief résumé of many of

Table 5.1 Daily kilocalories for maintenance of desirable weight;[10] the values below have been calculated for a moderately active person – someone who is very active should add on 50 kcal, and someone with a sedentary lifestyle should subtract 75 kcal

			Daily intake (kilocalories)					
Weight			Age 18–35 years		Age 35–55 years		Age 55–75 years	
St	lb	kg	Men	Women	Men	Women	Men	Women
7	1	44.9		1700		1500		1300
7	12	49.9	2200	1850	1950	1650	1650	1400
8	9	54.9	2400	2000	2150	1750	1850	1550
9	2	58.1		2100		1900		1600
9	6	59.9	2550	2150	2300	1950	1950	1650
10	3	64.9	2700	2300	2400	2050	2050	1800
11	0	69.9	2900	2400	2600	2150	2200	1850
11	11	74.8	3100	2550	2800	2300	2400	1950
12	8	79.8	3250		2950		2500	
13	5	84.8	3300		3100		2600	

the more common popular diets that people try as individuals, either informed by books or supported by private clinics or slimming clubs.

Some of these diets are not to be recommended, and they are included here for information only.

The breakfast-cereal diet[11]

Kellogg's cereal manufacturers had a terrific response to their 'two-week challenge' to lose about 2 kg in weight by replacing one meal a day with a bowl of cereal for a fortnight. Nutritionists from Queen Margaret University College in Edinburgh collaborated over the campaign. A total of 300 000 people have rung the Kellogg's helpline for advice, and 100 000 have visited Kellogg's website (www.kelloggs.com/products/cereals.html).

Most of the subjects who managed to achieve this weight loss maintained their weight loss by following a high-carbohydrate diet including plenty of potatoes, rice, pasta and bread.

The blood-group diet[12]

The theory behind this diet is that you should select a diet that matches your own blood group.

- Type O favours meat, fish and dairy products, whereas fruit, grains and vegetables should be eaten sparingly.
- Type A favours a vegetarian diet, including grains and fruit, whereas meat, wheat and dairy products should be avoided.
- Type B favours a mixed diet that includes meat, fish, vegetables, beans and fruit, whereas red meat, seeds and corn should be avoided.

The Atkins diet[12]

This is a high-protein, low-carbohydrate diet consisting of meat, cheese, etc., and avoiding starches, fruit, sugars and processed food.

Formula diet[13]

This is a balanced eating plan. The formula is to eat meals for which 40% of the calories are derived from carbohydrates, 30% are derived from protein and 30% from fats.

The Hay diet[14]

The Hay diet is also known as 'food combining for health'. It involves keeping starch foods separate from protein foods in order to aid digestion.

Weight-Watchers Pure Points[15]

Each person attending the Weight-Watchers weekly club session is privately weighed, and then there is a group discussion with the club leader to share news, hints and tips.

The 'Pure Points' programme allots points rather than calories to a variety of foods. Participants are allowed a predetermined number of points per day depending on how much they weigh and how much weight they need to lose. Most vegetables count as zero points, which means that participants can eat as many as they like. They can save points from their daily allowance to put towards a special food treat.

Weight-Watchers group members are encouraged to exercise and thus 'earn' extra points to spend on food. For instance, if they walk briskly for 30 minutes, they can add three points to their allowance.

Slimming Magazine clubs[15]

Each person attending the club meeting is weighed privately, and then the club leader gives a talk, after which there is an opportunity for those present to chat with each other. Each meeting has a particular theme. Non-members can attend a meeting before deciding whether to join the slimming club.

Slimming Magazine clubs have 18 eating plans, all of which are based on healthy eating guidelines. Each plan has a breakfast, lunch, main meal, snack, fruit allowance and an additional choice of calories. The 'Flexi' model is the most popular eating plan, and uses easy-to-prepare meals for the whole family. Other options include 'Little and Often', 'Back to Basics' and 'Vegetarian'.

Club members are encouraged to exercise and build more activity into their daily routines.

Rosemary Conley diet and fitness clubs[15]

Each person attending the meeting is weighed in private, and then an award is presented to the 'slimmer of the week'. After a five-minute talk on diet and nutrition, there is a physical activity workout for 45 minutes.

A popular low-fat diet option is called the 'New You Plan'. Club members are given a daily calorie allowance and allowed optional high-fat treats.

This is the only national slimming club in which members get dietary advice and exercise in the same class, although those attending do not have to do the workout if they do not want to join in.

Slimming World clubs[15]

Each person who attends the class is weighed in private. The class involves 'image therapy' to help give club members inspiration. The club offers lifelines – that is, access to consultants and other slimmers for support when members' willpower is low.

Club members choose between two diets – 'Original' and 'Green' – alternating between them as they like. The Green diet allows unlimited amounts of pasta, rice, potatoes, baked beans, pulses and grains. The Original diet permits unlimited lean meat, chicken, fish and seafood. Participants also eat three foods from the 'Healthy Extras' section each day to keep their diet balanced. In addition, they are allowed unlimited vegetables, most fruits and low-fat yogurts. They can also have 'sins' to splurge on 'naughtier' food which is high in fat and/or calories.

Those attending Slimming World clubs are encouraged to exercise in order to maximise their weight loss.

Low-fat diets

Many diets emphasise the reduction in fat intake which automatically reduces caloric intake, as fat is so high in calories. Very-low-calorie diets of around 800 kcal per day can induce rapid weight loss, but weight is often regained equally quickly once the diet has ceased. They are not generally recommended, but can be useful under medical supervision for specific reasons, such as the need for a patient to lose weight rapidly on medical grounds.[1,6]

Low-calorie diets

These are energy-restricted diets in the range 800–1500 kcal per day. They should contain a balance of protein, fat and carbohydrate, usually with reduced fat. Many of the diets described above fall within the category of a *low-calorie diet*.

High-dietary-fibre diets

Two studies that investigated the effects of dietary fibre found that fibre supplements were more effective than placebo when given with a diet of 1200–1600 kcal per day. However, the weight loss achieved was no different to that obtained with a comparable low-fibre/low-calorie diet.[16]

Very-low-calorie diets

This type of diet consists of 600 or 800 kcal or less per day. It is usually adopted for several days or weeks in order to achieve rapid weight loss. Lean muscle is lost as well as fat stores. Experts recommend a minimum protein intake of 0.8–1.5 g/kg of ideal body weight and daily vitamin and mineral supplements. Very-low-calorie diets should not be continued for more than four weeks.[6]

Decrease alcohol intake

Alcohol contains nearly as much energy as does fat, at 7 kcal/g. It can compromise a weight-reducing diet by providing hidden calories, and it is thought to alter the pattern of fat distribution, encouraging a 'beer belly'. Excessive amounts of alcohol act as a central depressant and sap initiative and willpower, reducing enthusiasm for physical exercise.

From compliance to concordance

When patients fail to comply with the terms of their prescribed medication the doctor or health professional usually feels let down. They may then restate the reasons why the patient should adhere to the recommended treatment, rather than explore the patient's health beliefs (culture, personality, family tradition and experience). The aim of concordance is to optimise health gain from the best use of medicines, with the patient's (weight) management being compatible with the approach that the patient desires and is capable of achieving.

This concept of concordance can be extrapolated from the situation of prescribing medicines for a health problem, to giving advice about lifestyle and weight management for those who are overweight or obese. The patient should be encouraged and enabled to communicate his or her health beliefs to the doctor or nurse, who should in turn communicate their professionally informed health beliefs to the patient and allow him or her to make as informed a choice as possible about the treatment, benefit and risk.

Box 5.2

An article by *Which* magazine (May 2001) has highlighted the potentially dangerous advice that many slimming books provide. High-protein/low-carbohydrate diets are criticised for their low fibre content, and for leaving the slimmer at risk of ketosis. The article pointed out the lack of evidence for the 'Hay' diet, in which proteins are not eaten at the same time as starch. Another criticism was that some diet books omit to state who the diets are suitable for, and who might suffer if they followed the diet described (e.g. children and people with diabetes).[17]

Reflection exercises

Exercise 8

Find out what initiatives have been undertaken by any of the practice team members to ascertain patients' views during the previous 12 months. This might have included surveying or involving anyone registered with the practice, including regular patients, people who do not use the services, carers, or people from the local community. How was the information that was gained from the initiative used? Did changes result? Your own or practice team members' learning needs from this exercise might include the following:

- learning more about the variety of methods that can be employed to find out patients' views – read up more on the subject[18]
- learning how to apply any of those methods to find out the views of people who are overweight or obese about the advice or treatment you offer for weight management, or what services they wish to receive
- learning more about organising a survey so that the findings are useful when making changes to the way in which services are planned or delivered, or the way in which staff behave (e.g. when a patient asks for a letter for a stairlift because of obesity)
- learning more about involving individual patients in decision making about the management of their weight (both initial weight control and sustaining weight loss).

Use these learning exercises to gather the views of overweight or obese individuals about one or more aspects of the way in which you provide care or services. Discuss the information you obtain with all of the relevant members of the practice team (*see* the worked example of a practice learning plan for ideas about whom you might involve), and plan how to make improvements in your services.

Exercise 9

Organise a tutorial with a dietitian. Hopefully you will have a community dietitian to whom you can refer your patients directly, but if not, choose one sited in the local hospital trust. Alternatively, invite the dietitian to come in to give a short teaching session to the practice team, or arrange to sit in with him or her on a typical clinic as an interested observer.

Your aim will be to try to find out 'what you didn't know you didn't know'. Best practice with regard to nutrition and diet is continually evolving as more research and development is undertaken and publicised. Therefore it is important to find a way to get up to date.

Exercise 10

Visit one or two local private slimming clubs to find out how they are run, and the theory behind their advice and information giving. Then you will feel more confident about signposting overweight or obese patients to the various clubs, and be able to reinforce sensible advice when patients return for follow-up appointments with you.

Now that you have completed these interactive reflection exercises, transfer the information to the empty template of the personal development plan on pages 141–151 if you are working on your own learning plan, or to the practice personal and professional development plan on pages 165–172 if you are working on a practice team learning plan. Don't forget to keep the evidence of your learning in your personal portfolio.

References

1 Scottish Intercollegiate Guidelines Network (SIGN) (1996) *Obesity in Scotland: integrating prevention with weight management.* SIGN, Edinburgh.

2 Royal College of Physicians of London (1998) *Clinical Management of Overweight and Obese Patients, With Particular Reference to the Use of Drugs.* Royal College of Physicians of London, London.

3 National Obesity Forum (2000) *NOF Guidelines for the Management of Obesity in Adults.* National Obesity Forum, Nottingham.

4 Wilding J (2000) Obesity. In: R Charlton (ed.) *Royal College of General Practitioners Members Reference Book 2000/2001.* Campden, London.

5 National Audit Office (2001) *Tackling Obesity in England.* National Audit Office, London.

6 Garrow J (chair) (1999) *Obesity. Report of the British Nutrition Foundation Task Force.* Blackwell Science, Oxford.

7 Hunt R, Rayner M and Sharp I (eds) (2000) *Health Update. Coronary heart disease and stroke.* Health Development Agency, London.

8 Cummings J and Bingham S (1998) Diet and the prevention of cancer. *BMJ.* **317**: 1636–40.

9 Food Standards Agency (1998) *Healthy Eating.* Food Standards Agency, London.

10 Medical Action Plan (1999) *Fat and Calorie Counter.* Harper Collins, Glasgow.

11 Wojtas O (2001) Why the academics weighed in with the ad men to confront a growing nutritional concern. *Times Higher Education Supplement.* **16 February**: 18–19.

12 Rignell M (2001) Types of diet. *She.* **March**: 31–2.

13 Daoust G and Daoust J (2001) Secrets of the fat. *Daily Mail.* **13 February**: 54–5.

14 Grant D and Joice J (1991) *Food Combining for Health. A new look at the Hay system.* Thorsons, London.

15 Norton S (2001) If you want to lose weight, join our club. *Family Circle.* **January**: 19–20.

16 Garrow J and Summerbell C (2002) Obesity. In: *Health Care Needs Assessment.* Third Series. Radcliffe Medical Press, Oxford.

17 Consumers' Association (2001) Ways to lose weight? *WHICH.* **May**: 34–37.

18 Chambers R (1999) *Involving Patients and the Public: how to do it better.* Radcliffe Medical Press, Oxford.

CHAPTER 6

Alternative approaches: behavioural therapy, physical activity and other techniques

Behavioural treatment is used to intervene in behaviour that is learned and reinforced by social circumstances – this is very relevant to people who overeat. Research has shown that adult behaviour change needs to be reinforced every five years.[1]

Behavioural therapy has a place in all three of the objectives of treatment of people with established obesity:

1 to assist the person in achieving a weight at which the health risks of obesity are reduced to the lowest possible level for that individual
2 to help the person to maintain this weight loss indefinitely
3 to maintain or restore the person's self-esteem if necessary.[2]

Box 6.1

'A combination of advice on diet and exercise, supported by behaviour therapy, is probably more effective than either diet or exercise advice alone in the treatment of obesity, and might lead to sustained weight loss.'[3]

Behavioural treatments alone do not seem to be effective in tackling obesity, and they should be used in combination with other approaches. A behavioural approach such as a person charting their daily weight can effectively reinforce other behavioural therapies. For example, long-term follow-up of patients who have received cognitive behavioural therapy has shown that the initial 5–10% weight loss that is usually achieved rarely persists, and that they gradually return to their original weight. The combination of cognitive behavioural therapy,

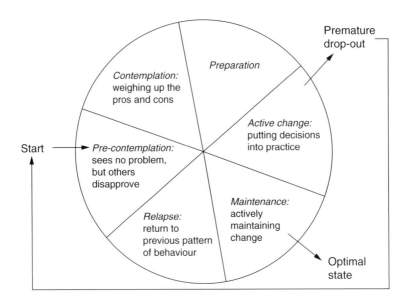

good nutrition and a reasonable amount of exercise offers more hope of achieving a sustained weight loss.[3,4]

Any behavioural approach should take into account the fact that eating is a highly reinforcing behaviour. It induces feelings of gratification and pleasure which for some people is their main source of pleasure, and such individuals will not forsake their 'eating for pleasure' habit very readily.

We need to avoid medicalising obesity by applying stringent guidelines to weight management, and to look for new ways of tackling obesity as a society.

In order to understand what intervention to use to try to help patients to lose weight, you need to determine whether each individual is ready to change, to conquer their overweight or obesity and to sustain that weight loss. Then you can match your approach or intervention to the stage at which they are at present.

The five stages of change are illustrated in Figure 6.1 above. They include the following:

1   *pre-contemplation*: 'the stage at which there is no intention to change behaviour in the foreseeable future'
2   *contemplation*: 'the stage at which people are aware that a problem exists and are seriously thinking about overcoming it, but have not yet made a commitment to take action'
3   *preparation*: 'the stage that combines intention and behavioural criteria; individuals at this stage are intending to take action in

the next month, and may have unsuccessfully taken action in the past year'

4 *active change*: 'the stage at which individuals modify their behaviour, experiences or environment in order to overcome their problems'.

5 *maintenance*: 'the stage at which people work to prevent relapse and consolidate the gains attained during the action'.[5]

Types of behavioural therapy[1,4]

Cognitive behaviour programme

This includes traditional cognitive behavioural approaches such as the following:

- self-monitoring (e.g. keeping a diary of food eaten and the calorie and/ or fat content)
- stimulus control – developing strategies for an individual to reduce exposure to stimuli which may trigger inappropriate eating
- coping with cravings and high-risk situations
- stress management, especially for those who report stress-induced eating behaviour
- relaxation techniques
- learned self-control – breaking the cycle between certain stimuli to eating particular foods and eating inappropriately
- problem-solving skills.

Other approaches with relevance to weight-loss management include the following:

- healthy eating advice, and modification of disordered eating patterns (e.g. working with someone who is 'binge eating', to encourage a normal eating pattern)
- weight management – setting behavioural goals that reflect changes in eating behaviour or exercise habits
- mood management
- managing work and family
- relapse prevention – various mechanisms so that the individual accepts that lapses are to be expected and understands how they might avoid a 'relapse'
- avoiding self-defeating thinking (e.g. 'all-or-nothing' thinking)
- improving body image – learning to dissociate body image and self-esteem.

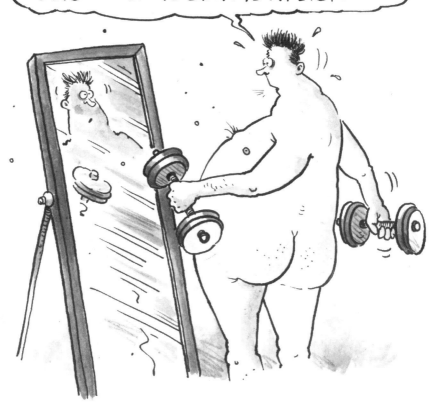

Behavioural choice treatment

This refers to a cognitive behavioural intervention based on a decision-making model for an individual person's food choice. The outcomes and goals associated with food choice include self-esteem and social acceptance.

Standard behaviour therapy

This is a behavioural weight-management programme that employs moderate calorie restriction to promote weight loss.

Avoiding situations that tempt the person to overeat may be more effective than behavioural approaches that involve role play, where the participant practises resisting overeating or social pressures to overeat.

Box 6.1 Issues to be tackled in group behavioural therapy[6]

- The importance of self-monitoring using a food diary.
- The need for a long-term lifestyle change.
- The need to modify eating habits in order to lose weight.
- Assessing how much exercise is currently taken and how to increase this.
- Restricting occasions and situations when inappropriate types or amounts of food (or alcohol) are consumed.
- Separating eating from other activities.
- Planning daily food intake.
- Adapting recipes with regard to fat, fibre, salt and sugar content.
- Identifying causes of negative emotions and stress.
- Recognising when eating is used as a way of coping with stress.
- Finding ways of coping with stress as alternatives to eating.
- Understanding how to deal with situations that interfere with everyday food choice at work, at home and socially.

Interventions that increase physical activity in sedentary people

There are many health benefits of physical activity in people who are obese.[7] They include the following:

- a favourable modification of blood lipids
- a reduction in blood pressure, even in the absence of weight loss
- improved management or prevention of type 2 diabetes mellitus
- improved functional capacity, which is typically low in the obese
- reductions in mild clinical depression and anxiety (both of which are common in people who are obese)
- improved self-esteem and general psychological well-being.

Physical activity increases energy output, enhances fat loss and prevents weight gain. It also serves to reduce cardiovascular risk factors and increase personal motivation, confidence and self-esteem. Attitudes often need to be challenged in order to enable patients to begin to enjoy physical activity, find the time to be active and decrease the amount of time spent in sedentary activity. Patients should be encouraged to write down their feelings about exercise and diet in their progress diary, and to try to recognise any emotional triggers that make them eat.[8]

The health benefits from an exercise promotion intervention can persist over a long period of time. In one research trial in which women were followed up ten years later, those who had been encouraged to walk at the start of the study reported significantly more walking than those who had not been encouraged to walk.[4] Similarly, in another study of women aged over 80 years, women who had received home visits from a physiotherapist were significantly more active after one year than those who had received social visits. In total, 42% of those who had been advised by the physiotherapist were still completing the recommended exercise programme at least three times a week. The intervention was also shown to decrease the risk of falling in those in the exercise group.[4]

Box 6.3 Posters can prompt less active people to use the stairs[9]

Using the stairs instead of the lift is a relatively painless way to increase physical activity. When posters urging people to use the stairs rather than the lift were displayed in a shopping mall, less active shoppers responded well to the message. Pre-contemplators (i.e. those not considering changing to a more active lifestyle) were less likely to notice the posters than those at other stages in the cycle of change (*see* page 84). Defaulters most often stated that it was easier to take the lift or that they were too lazy to use the stairs. The authors of the study suggest that physical health promotion should address motivational barriers to stair climbing.

Behavioural modification can be helpful in the promotion of physical activity. Ask patients to keep a daily diary and plan physical activity for the following day, and then confirm that it has been done. Encourage patients to build up the time they spend being active, and to find more active ways of doing their normal activities (e.g. by making leisure pursuits more active).[1]

Exercise referral schemes recognise that many people do not like using gyms or other special sports facilities, or that they find them inconvenient. The philosophy of such schemes is to provide an educational experience that motivates people to be more active in the long term – for example, by walking or cycling.[10]

Box 6.4

One general practice in South Staffordshire worked jointly with the parish council to publish information about local walks for the patient population as self-help booklets. Nurses targeted appropriate patients with cardiovascular disease to encourage them to join in 'practice walks'.

Wharf Surgery, Gnosall, South Staffordshire

Local authorities and health authorities are expected to organise programmes to promote exercise. These may involve employers and workplaces, the educational sector (including schools or colleges), and transport and leisure services (to create cycle paths or safer walking areas) or community groups. The types of interventions to which those in primary care might be expected to contribute include the following:

• individual patient risk assessment and advice – identifying current activity levels and introducing suitable interventions
• counselling with regard to behaviour change – encouraging patients to develop their own strategies for becoming more active
• exercise referral – to a recognised scheme with qualified staff (e.g. leisure professionals)
• promoting the use of local leisure facilities
• encouraging community-based 'health walks'.[7,10]

Box 6.5 Energy expenditure associated with non-exercise activity[11]

Sitting and fidgeting uses a third more energy than lying motion-less. Standing and fidgeting uses nearly twice as much energy as standing motionless, although the exact amount of energy expended varies between individuals. Fidgeting for 2.5 hours can work off as much as 200 kilocalories.

The Internet can help – or harm

Box 6.6

A group of hospital employees successfully lost weight using an Internet program that sent them regular emails. Half of the group were put on a six-month programme of Internet education and the other half were put on a programme of Internet behavioural therapy. All of the participants had a face-to-face weight loss session, and had access to a website. Those who received behavioural therapy were sent weekly behavioural lessons via email, and had to submit weekly diaries. The group who received behavioural therapy lost more weight and showed a greater decrease in waist circumference.[12]

However, there are potential hazards associated with using the Internet indiscriminately, as the report in Box 6.7 illustrates.

Box 6.7 Potential hazards associated with obtaining information from the Internet[13]

According to recent evidence, the general public should beware of the plethora of unsound advice about dieting if they trawl the Internet for advice or buy products to aid slimming.

About one million links were retrieved by search engines, of which 50 links were evaluated. Three links gave sound dietary advice, 11 links offered dietary replacements and 15 links offered vitamin, herbal or mineral supplements. Typically, the pro-grammes recommended that two meals per day should be replaced by protein drinks, and the third meal should be restricted to

400 calories. Meaningless terms abounded. The advice available ranged from totally sound to dubious, misleading and downright dangerous.

However, the Health Education Board for Scotland is an example of a good Internet site. It offers dependable advice on healthy eating, and can be recommended to patients at www.hebs.scot.nhs.uk.

Acupuncture

There is no evidence that acupuncture aids weight loss. However, it is practised with this intention, and there are anecdotal reports that attribute success in losing weight to acupuncture.

This approach should always be combined with dietary advice. The acupuncturist attempts to diagnose any psychological cause, such as insecurity, depression or loneliness, and to individualise their treatment accordingly. One of the recommended sites is the ear, and the acupuncture needle might be inserted in the stomach, hunger and *shenmen* points in the ear for 15–20 minutes. Additional acupuncture body points can be used during the same treatment session to exert a calming and balancing effect on the body, or to stimulate organs that are thought to be deficient in energy.[14]

Strategies to maintain weight loss

Most people begin to regain weight a few months after ceasing to actively lose it, so strategies to maintain weight loss are important.

The more personal contact there is with a therapist over time, the less likely it is for weight gain to occur, and the more likely it is that there will be greater weight loss. Two-weekly contact with the patient seems to be the optimal frequency for providing support.[6] In addition, self-help peer groups, self-management techniques or family/spouse support may also increase weight loss. The largest weight loss occurred when multiple strategies were employed.[4]

A group setting helps most patients to achieve more weight loss than if they are being seen individually by a professional, although some men with severe obesity maintain their weight loss better by individual management.[6]

The evidence as to whether frequent telephone contact, continued self-monitoring or urge control reduces the rate of weight regain is inconclusive. One intervention that has been tried is low-intensity education with a financial incentive to maintain weight compared with an untreated control group. There was a significantly greater average weight loss in the intervention group compared with the control group. However, other research that trialled low-intensity education via a mailed newsletter with and without a financial incentive found no difference between the average weight gained by the study groups over a three-year period.[4] There is concern that even if we identify successful strategies, anything other than those of low intensity will not be affordable on a wide scale.

Reflection exercises

Exercise 11

Visit a neighbouring practice and compare the way in which you manage overweight and obesity in your patients with their systems and procedures. Compare your practice protocols for the management of overweight and obesity, and coronary heart disease as a whole, while you are there. Focus particularly on behavioural therapies and promoting physical activity, as in this chapter. Look for gaps in your protocols of which you were previously unaware, and refine your protocols accordingly.

Exercise 12

Visit one or two local private and local authority-owned sports centres to find out how they are run, what facilities they offer (e.g. individual training and group classes) and their general approach to physical activity. Then you will feel more confident about sign-posting overweight or obese patients to the various clubs and be able to reinforce sensible advice when patients return for follow-up appointments with you. You will learn about any rules that the various clubs or centres maintain about taking responsibility for people with various medical conditions, including obesity, without involving health professionals in certifying them as 'fit' to participate.

Exercise 13

Review how well your behavioural strategies are working to aid over-weight or obese patients in losing weight. Discuss this with other members of the practice team over coffee. Do they have any informal feedback or suggestions about how your current practice is working or new approaches that you and other team members could try?

Try to detect that behavioural approaches you use work better than others in motivating overweight or obese patients to reduce their weight, and why these individuals have not controlled their weight in the past. Next time you advise someone to keep a self-monitoring food and activity diary, give them a short evaluation form to complete about how it works out for them. Collate several evaluation forms and look for any patterns. Target a specific patient group (e.g. those with diabetes) where you know you will be reviewing patients every few months and the audit or review will be more easily arranged.

Now that you have completed these interactive reflection exercises, transfer the information to the empty template of the personal development plan on pages 141–151 if you are working on your own learning plan, or to the practice personal and professional development plan on pages 165–172 if you are working on a practice team learning plan. Don't forget to keep the evidence of your learning in your personal portfolio.

References

1 Wardle J (1999) Treatment of obesity. IV. Behavioural treatment. In: *Obesity. The Report of the British Nutrition Foundation Task Force.* Blackwell Science, Oxford.

2 Garrow J and Summerbell C (2002) Obesity. In: *Health Care Needs Assessment.* Third Series. Radcliffe Medical Press, Oxford.

3 NHS Centre for Reviews and Dissemination (1997) The prevention and treatment of obesity. *Effect Health Care Bull.* **3**: 1–12.

4 Barton S (ed.) (2001) *Clinical Evidence. Issue 5.* BMJ Publishing, London.

5 Prochaska J, DiClemente C and Norcross J (1992) In search of how people change: applications to addictive behaviours. *Am Psychol.* **47**: 1102–11.

6 Scottish Intercollegiate Guidelines Network (SIGN) (1996) *Obesity in Scotland: integrating prevention with weight management.* SIGN, Edinburgh.

7 Hunt R, Rayner M and Sharp I (eds) (2000) *Health Update: coronary heart disease and stroke.* Health Development Agency, London.

8 Medical Action Plan (1999) *Fat and Calorie Counter.* Harper Collins, Glasgow.

9 Kerr J, Eves F and Carroll D (2000) Posters can prompt less active people to use the stairs. *J Epidemiol Commun Health.* **54**: 942–3.

10 Department of Health (2001) *Exercise Referral Systems: a national quality framework.* Department of Health, London; www.doh.gov.uk/exercise referrals.

11 Levine J, Schleusner SJ and Jensen MD (2000) Energy expenditure of nonexercise activity. *Am J Clin Nutr.* **72**: 1451–4.

12 Tate DF (2001) Using internet technology to deliver a behavioural weight loss program. *JAMA.* **285**: 1172–7.

13 Miles J, Petrie C and Steel M (2000) Slimming on the Internet. *J R Soc Med.* **93**: 254–7.

14 Ross J (1995) *Acupuncture Point Combinations.* Churchill Livingstone, Edinburgh.

CHAPTER 7

Drug therapy for obesity

David Haslam

In 1903 the makers of *Antipon,* described as the 'King of Corpulence Cures', made the following claims for their product:[1]

- 'permanent elegance and sounder health are the priceless gifts conferred by a short economical and pleasant course of Antipon'
- 'within a day and a night of taking the first dose there will be a reduction of weight of up to 3 lb or even more'
- 'contains no injurious substances'
- 'without perfect health there is no physical beauty, and in giving back the one, Antipon assures the other'
- 'no irksome dietary restrictions to observe; the subject eats heartily'
- 'a permanent cure; it destroys the tendency to excessive fat development'.

Antipon was analysed in 1909 by the British Medical Association in an attempt to rationalise drug treatment and expose fraudulent claims for therapeutic substances. It was found to contain nothing more than citric acid diluted with alcohol, water and colouring. Nevertheless, Antipon sold extremely well at two shillings and sixpence per bottle, more as a tribute to the power of advertising than to medical science.[2]

However, just such a magical drug which bestows permanent beauty, grace, elegance and slimness upon its user without the need to diet or exercise is still what some patients expect when they present to the doctor's surgery.

Pharmacotherapy

Drug therapy for obesity is a second-line treatment for selected patients in whom dietary measures, exercise regimes and behavioural therapy have proved inadequate. It may only be offered as an adjunct to other forms of treatment.

Patient selection

Drug therapy is considered to be appropriate for patients with either a BMI of 30 kg/m² or more, or a BMI of 28 kg/m² or more in the presence of significant comorbidities (e.g. ischaemic heart disease or diabetes), and such prescription is within the remit of the drug's licence.[3–5]

Alternative forms of management, including supervised dietary restriction, lifestyle and behavioural therapy, should be attempted for a period of at least three months before initiating drug therapy. If this achieves a reduction in body weight of 10% and weight loss is continuing, then drug treatment should be avoided or postponed (*see* section below for specific guidance on the use of orlistat).[3–5]

Before deciding that drug therapy is justified, the treating clinician should consider the following:

- the risks to an individual of continuing obesity
- the comorbid risk factors or complications from obesity
- the balance between the health benefits of maintained weight and the potential adverse effects of the drug, if weight loss has stopped.[1]

Aims of drug treatment

The aims of drug therapy are to reduce mortality and morbidity associated with obesity. In common with first-line treatments, the target of a 10% maintained weight reduction is a realistic and attainable ambition. The presence of certain comorbidities (e.g. severe osteo-arthritis or ischaemic heart disease) may render exercise and exertion impossible, and the likelihood of losing weight may seem to be negligible. Drug management can help to break this vicious circle by initiating weight loss, and allowing more freedom of movement and exertion and a healthier lifestyle.

Maintenance of weight loss *can* be achieved in the medium term (e.g. for one year) by continuing drug therapy. Beyond that, weight maintenance relies on permanent lifestyle changes.

Choice of drugs

Most of the anti-obesity drugs that have been used in the past have been withdrawn because they are ineffective or have adverse effects.

Drugs should never be used as the sole element of treatment – other components of managed care should continue. Drug treatment should be discontinued if weight loss is less than 5% after the first 12 weeks, or if the patient gains weight at any time while they are receiving drug treatment.[6]

Combination therapy involving more than one anti-obesity drug is contraindicated.

Drugs that act on the gastrointestinal tract

Bulking agents

These are agents such as methylcellulose and ispaghula husk, which are used to induce a feeling of fullness of the stomach. However, there is no evidence that they are beneficial in the long-term treatment of overweight and obesity. Patients should be told to take plenty of water with the tablets, as the latter swell when in contact with liquid, and not to take them before going to bed.

Pancreatic lipase inhibitor (orlistat)[3,6–10]

Orlistat inhibits fat breakdown in the lumen of the stomach and the small intestine. It inhibits pancreatic and gastric lipases and works by decreasing the hydrolysis of ingested triglycerides, thus reducing dietary fat absorption by around one-third. People who take orlistat excrete about 32% of ingested fat in their faeces, compared with 4.4% in controls. This leads to greater and more rapid weight loss.

Orlistat is used as an adjunct to dietary, lifestyle and behavioural therapies in patients with sufficient motivation to adhere to an appropriate dietary regime. It is used in conjunction with a mildly hypocaloric diet with around one-third of the calories supplied by fat. Orlistat has an optimum effect at a dose of 120 mg three times a day. It is taken before, during, or up to an hour after each main meal, and the dose is omitted if a meal is missed or contains no fat.[6]

Box 7.1 Criteria for prescribing orlistat[7]

- The licensing criteria and the National Institute for Clinical Excellence (NICE) recommendations require potential patients to lose 2.5 kg in the month preceding the first prescription for orlistat. This enables treating doctors to ascertain whether a person is able to maintain a suitably low fat intake and a reasonable amount of physical activity.
- Patients should have documented evidence of a BMI of 30 or above (and no significant comorbidity necessarily) or a BMI of 28 or above with significant comorbidity (e.g. diabetes, hypertension or dyslipidaemia).
- Patients taking orlistat should be monitored and weighed on a monthly basis thereafter as part of a supervised weight management plan.
- Patients who are continuing to be prescribed orlistat should show a 5% weight loss three months after the start of drug treatment and at least a 10% cumulative weight loss six months after the start of treatment.
- Orlistat can only be prescribed for adults aged 18 to 75 years.

Orlistat is not absorbed from the gastrointestinal tract, so there are minimal systemic side-effects. As there is reduced absorption of the fat-soluble vitamins, including vitamins A and D, vitamin supplements may be required. There is no evidence of a link between orlistat and breast cancer, which was originally listed as a possible side-effect. The drug is contraindicated in pregnancy and whilst breastfeeding, and for patients with cholestasis and malabsorption syndromes.

As a result of the decreased fat absorption from the bowel, the increased fat content of the faeces gives rise to dark-coloured oily stools, in contrast to the pale offensive stools associated with steator-rhoea in pancreatic disorders. The faecal fat content is usually negligible with a low- or moderate-fat diet, but if an inappropriately high level of fat is ingested, then extremely fatty stools with oily discharge, urgency, flatulence, soiling and even faecal incontinence can occur with associated abdominal pain. This serves to reinforce dietary and behavioural advice, hopefully leading to the introduction of a lower-fat diet rather than abandonment of the restricted diet regime.

Several research trials have demonstrated the effectiveness of orlistat. The percentage weight loss was greater in patients on orlistat and a mildly hypocaloric diet (500–800 kcal/day deficit) compared with those taking a placebo drug and a similar diet.[8,9] In a two-year study of 688 patients, those taking orlistat lost an average 10% of their ideal body weight by the end of the first year on a hypocaloric diet, compared with 6% of those on placebo. In total, 39% of those in the orlistat group lost more than 10% of their ideal body weight, compared with 18% of those taking a placebo. The patients who received orlistat during year 1 were then randomised to receive orlistat or a placebo in year 2, together with a eucaloric diet. Those taking orlistat regained an average of 26% of the weight lost, compared with an average of 43% in the patients who had taken a placebo in year 2.[9]

There is some evidence that orlistat helps to reduce the risks associated with comorbidities.[9–12] In one study, those taking orlistat showed significant improvements in the form of reduced levels of total and LDL-cholesterol, fasting plasma glucose and blood pressure.[8] Other studies have confirmed these findings, demonstrating improved glycaemic control, with a reduction in HbA_{1c} and dyslipidaemias in those with type 2 diabetes.[10–13]

Centrally acting drugs

Centrally acting drugs act on serotoninergic or noradrenergic pathways, or both. In recent years many of these drugs have been withdrawn from use because of the incidence of side-effects. Fenfluramine and the combination of phentermine with dexfenfluramine have been withdrawn because of their link with heart valve defects.

Sibutramine

Sibutramine creates a feeling of satiety by acting as a serotonin and noradrenaline reuptake inhibitor in the brain, with the result that patients feel satisfied after eating smaller quantities of food. It may also increase thermogenesis by a stimulant action on the peripheral noradrenergic system. The dose of 10 mg once daily is well absorbed from the stomach and has a half-life of 14–16 hours. It is mainly excreted in the urine. There is limited evidence that sibutramine can increase weight loss compared with placebo in healthy adults with BMI values of 27 to 40 kg/m.[2] This weight loss was not sustained over time or after stopping treatment.[8] Weight loss is maximal during the first six months and continues at a slower rate thereafter.[14,15]

Specific studies have highlighted the benefits of sibutramine-induced weight loss in people who are obese and have hypertension, diabetes, hyperlipidaemia and/or other comorbidities. Sibutramine can reduce the level of total cholesterol and triglycerides, with an increase in HDL cholesterol levels, and can improve glycaemic control in type 2 diabetes.[16,17]

A 24-week study of 175 obese patients with poorly controlled type 2 diabetes showed that those individuals on sibutramine lost significantly greater amounts of weight and percentages of their ideal body weight than controls, when on a moderately hypocaloric diet. Patients on sibutramine lost an average of 4.3 kg or 4.5% of their ideal body weight, whilst those on placebo lost an average of 0.4 kg or 0.5% of their ideal body weight. A weight loss of more than 5% occurred in one-third of patients taking sibutramine, but none of those individuals who were taking a placebo lost 5% of their body weight. Patients who lost weight also benefited from reduced HbA_{1c} and fasting glucose levels, an improved lipid profile and a better quality of life.[16]

Another study of 127 patients over a period of 12 weeks concluded that sibutramine, 10 mg once daily, is a useful and effective therapy for obesity in those with stable hypertension. Weight reduction averaged 4.4 kg in patients taking sibutramine, compared with 2.2 kg for the placebo group. A reduction in body weight was associated with a reduction in blood pressure in both treatment and control groups.[17]

Common side-effects of sibutramine include headache, dry mouth, constipation, anorexia, insomnia, rhinitis and pharyngitis in 10–30% of patients. A small mean increase in mean blood pressure of 1–2 mmHg is observed in patients on sibutramine, and an average increase in heart rate of 4–5 beats per minute.[4]

Phentermine

Phentermine is an appetite suppressant with stimulant qualities, which can lead to a modest weight loss in the medium term in people who are more than 15% overweight, when associated with a restricted calorie diet. However, there tends to be rapid weight regain on withdrawal of the drug. The severe side-effect of pulmonary hypertension is uncommon. Adverse reactions such as dry mouth and headache are more common, and the drug can lead to dependence.

It is given in a dose of 15–30 mg daily for 12 weeks or less. Phentermine is not recommended for the routine management of obesity, and is categorised in *Clinical Evidence* as 'likely to be ineffective or harmful'.[6,8]

Fluoxetine

There is limited and conflicting evidence that the selective serotonin reuptake inhibitor fluoxetine has any beneficial effect on obesity. It is neither licensed nor recommended for this purpose.[8]

Unsuitable drugs for the treatment of obesity

Diuretics, purgatives, hormone treatments (including human chorionic gonadotrophin and dehydroepiandrosterone (DHEA)), ephedrine, amphetamines and amphetamine-like substances are unsuitable for the treatment of obesity. Certain compounds are an appropriate part of obesity management in the presence of coexisting conditions (e.g. thyroxine in cases of biochemically-proven hypothyroidism, metformin and acarbose in the presence of non-insulin-dependent diabetes).

History of over-the-counter remedies

The history of the treatment of 'corpulence' is littered with 'such regimens as bleeding, blistering, purging, starving, the use of different kinds of baths, and of drugs innumerable, most of which have been found utterly to fail in accomplishing the desired object'. Cynics would claim that very little has changed.[18]

Antacid draughts and alkalis have been used for centuries because of the 'chemical affinity of the alkalis for fats'. They probably did less harm than other cures such as the *Motherby Mercurial Remedy* and *Dr Harcourt's Arsenite of Potassa*, which included among its side-effects 'a gradual sinking of the powers of life; a nameless feeling of illness, failure of the strength, an aversion to food and drink and to all enjoyments of life' as well as being 'destructive to animal and vegetable life'.[18]

For many years *citric acid* was widely believed to have slimming powers. The Marquis of Cortona, 'by drinking vinegar, reduced his body from a condition of enormous obesity so that he could fold his skin about him like a garment'. However, rather than illustrating any beneficial slimming powers attributable to vinegar, this demonstrates its 'pernicious powers on the health'. Even more unpalatable was the remedy proposed by Dr Thomas Short in 1728 who, noting the power of soap to emulsify fats, recommended its use both externally and internally by those who 'labour involuntarily under the Incumbrances of Flesh and Blood'.

The ancient and historical remedies with the best credentials were based on herbal and other botanical substances, many of which are still available and widely used.

Herbal/alternative and botanical remedies

Herbal, botanical and other natural remedies for obesity have been used in various cultures for centuries.

Nicholas Culpeper, the seventeenth-century English herbalist recommended a number of therapies, including fennel ('Both Leaves, Seeds and Roots hereof are much used in Drinks or Broths, to make people more spare and lean that are too fat') and ash ('The Water distilled therefrom, being taken a small quantity every morning fasting, is a singular Medicine for those that are subject to a Dropsie, or to abate the greatness of those who are too gross or fat').

The medicinal powers of *Fucus vesiculosus*, better known as bladderwrack (a type of seaweed), have been used to treat corpulence for hundreds of years, and if Victorian textbooks and nineteenth-century editions of the *British Medical Journal* are to believed, it had a remarkable success rate. The 1894 edition of the *Extra Pharmacopoeia* informs us that 'Preparations of this seaweed, being rich in iodine, bromine and chlorine salts, have for a long time had the reputation of being useful in treating corpulence in a dosage of 1 or 2 drachms before meals'. Its action was thought to relate to the stimulation of the thyroid gland and the subsequent effect on the metabolic rate, but it also has diuretic properties. In 1879, *The Practitioner* reported a case in which fucus, 'combined with liquor potassae, reduced the fat of a lad who had suddenly become very corpulent'. The *British Medical Journal* of the same year relates the story of 'a lady who lost 20 lb in 9 weeks when taking the liquid extract, without bad results'. However, some doubt was cast by contemporaries who observed that the same extract was being used simultaneously to fatten pigs in Ireland![19]

Fucus vesiculosus is still being used as a treatment for obesity, either on its own or in combination with other substances such as ginseng.[20] Other popular herbal remedies include angelica, capsicum, cleavers, dropwort, Irish moss, Poke root, sassafras and many others. Some remedies cause weight loss because of their purgative or diuretic properties (e.g. senna and cascara, which can be found in various concoctions). Ephedra, known as 'Herbal Ecstasy', from which ephedrine is derived, has sympathomimetic properties and is controversially marketed as an obesity cure despite its well-documented risks. Some of these substances undoubtedly cause a degree of weight loss, but there is no convincing scientific evidence to suggest that any herbal or botanical remedies have a place in the long-term treatment of obesity.

An Indian remedy that is renowned for aiding weight loss is *gugulipid*, which has been used for centuries to treat lipid disorders and obesity, and is said to mediate its effects through thyroid stimulation.

Griffonia simplicifolia is an African plant from which commercial quantities of serotonin are extracted.

Each year a new crop of obesity remedies is touted as the best ever, long-awaited panacea. Much pseudoscience is published to support these claims. Compounds such as the 'fountain of youth hormone' DHEA, pyruvate, fat-magnets, slimming patches, lipotropic substances, and various amino acids have been endorsed by scientific institutions, backed up by anecdotal case histories and testimonials. However, there is no convincing scientific evidence to support their efficacy.

Long-term follow-up after drug treatment

Patients who are prescribed anti-obesity drugs should be supervised at least monthly, and a record should be kept of their body weight, blood pressure, etc., as appropriate.[1]

Programmes for weight management should continue after drug therapy has ceased in order to try to prevent rebound weight regain. It is possible to continue anti-obesity drugs in the medium term to achieve this aim, but the permanent nature of dietary and lifestyle changes should be monitored on a regular basis (e.g. 3 to 6-monthly) after withdrawal of treatment.

Once a weight-loss target has been achieved and maintained, consider negotiating a new target. This may involve re-establishing a drug regime.[1]

Research

Current research in the field of drug therapy for obesity includes studies on leptin, the 'fat hormone', beta-3-adrenoceptors, cholecystokinin boosters, neuropeptide Y antagonists and growth hormone.

Reflection exercises

Exercise 14

Review the case notes of 10 patients identified as obese and look at the treatment they have been given (pharmacological or psychological). How does it compare with the best practice described in this chapter on drug therapy?

If you have classified patients by Read coding (*see* page 24) and can identify 10 patients who are obese, then undertake an audit of those case notes. If you do not have such a computerised system, see how many patients you can recall, and ask other practice colleagues whom they can remember. Reviewing 10 patients' notes should give you an indication of how well you are doing as an individual or as a practice.

If you cannot identify 10 patients from computerised records, is the institution of computerised records with comprehensive information about risk factors a learning need for you or others in your practice team?

Exercise 15

Find all the patient literature that you have in your practice for people who are overweight or obese. Does the literature match the most up-to-date thinking about best practice in weight management? Or does it promote out-of-date practices and approaches or use old terminology? You will need to be clear yourself what the most up-to-date recommendations are in order to be able to check your literature and complete this exercise.

Now that you have completed these interactive reflection exercises, transfer the information to the empty template of the personal development plan on pages 141–151 if you are working on your own learning plan, or to the practice personal and professional development plan on pages 165–172 if you are working on a practice team learning plan. Don't forget to keep the evidence of your learning in your personal portfolio.

References

1 Antipon advertisements appeared in *The Illustrated London News*, 21 November 1903, 4 August 1906 and 8 December 1906.

2 British Medical Association (1909) *Secret Remedies. What they cost and what they contain.* British Medical Association, London.

3 McNeely W and Benfield P (1998) Orlistat. *Drugs.* **56**:241–9.

4 Kopelman P (chair) (1998) *Clinical Management of Overweight and Obese Patients.* Royal College of Physicians of London, London.

5 Kopelman P (1999) Treatment of obesity. V. Pharmacotherapy for obesity. In: *Obesity. Report of the British Nutrition Foundation Task Force.* Blackwell Science, Oxford.

6 Joint Formulary Committee (2001) *British National Formulary.* British Medical Association and Royal Pharmaceutical Society of Great Britain, London.

7 National Institute for Clinical Excellence (2001) *Guidance on the Use of Orlistat for the Treatment of Obesity in Adults.* National Institute for Clinical Excellence, London.

8 Barton S (ed.) (2001) *Clinical Evidence. Issue 5.* BMJ Publishing, London.

9 Sjostrom L, Rissanen A, Andersen T *et al.* (1998) Randomised placebo-controlled trial of orlistat for weight loss and prevention of weight regain in obese patients. *Lancet.* **352**: 167–72.

10 Rossner S, Sjostrom L, Noack R *et al.* (2000) Weight loss, weight maintenance and improved cardiovascular risk factors after 2 years of treatment with orlistat for obesity. *Obesity Res.* **8**: 49–61.

11 Zavoral JH (1998) Treatment with orlistat reduces cardiovascular risk in obese patients. *J Hypertension.* **16**: 2013–17.

12 Hollander PA, Elbein SC, Hirsch IB *et al.* (1998) Role of orlistat in the treatment of obese patients with type 2 diabetes. *Diabetes Care.* **21**: 1288–94.

13 Heymsfield SB, Segal KR, Hauptman J *et al.* (2000) Effects of weight loss with orlistat on glucose tolerance and progression to type 2 diabetes in obese adults. *Arch Intern Med.* **19**: 1321–6.

14 Bray GA, Blackburn GL, Ferguson JM *et al.* (1999) Sibutramine produces dose-related weight loss. *Obesity Res.* **7**: 189–98.

15 Apfelbaum M, Vague P, Ziegler O *et al.* (1999) Long-term maintenance of weight loss after a very low calorie diet: a randomised trial of the efficacy and tolerability of sibutramine. *Am J Med.* **106**: 179–84.

16 Fujioka K, Seaton TB, Rowe E *et al.* and the Sibutramine/Diabetes Clinical Study Group (2000) Weight loss with sibutramine improves glycaemic

control and other metabolic parameters in obese patients with type 2 diabetes. *Diabetes Obesity Metab.* **2**: 175–8.

17 Sjostrum L, Rissanen A, Andersen T *et al.* for the European Multicentre Orlistat Study Group (2000) Randomized double-blind placebo-controlled multicenter study of sibutramine in obese hypertensive patients. *Cardiology.* **94**: 152–8.

18 Russell FC (1894) *Corpulency and the Cure.* Woburn House, London.

19 Hart E (ed.) (1879) Extra Pharmacopoeia. *BMJ.* **2**: 482.

20 Fetrow C and Avila J (1999) *Complementary and Alternative Medicines.* Springhouse, Pennsylvania.

CHAPTER 8

Surgical treatments for obesity

David Haslam

Surgery is a treatment option in severely obese individuals in whom non-surgical treatment has failed, and who have consented to surgery following thorough assessment, screening and counselling. Bariatric surgery is an extremely effective method for long-term weight management once non-invasive approaches have failed.[1] ('Bariatrics' is the term given to that branch of medicine which involves the management of obesity.) Surgery for obesity is more effective than other modalities in maintaining weight loss.

Weight-reduction surgery can only be considered for a tiny minority of patients once all other treatment options have been exhausted. There are operative risks as well as financial costs.

Such surgery can result in massive weight loss. A review of eight randomised controlled trials[2] reported on the extent of weight loss from surgical intervention in individuals with a BMI of $40 \, \text{kg/m}^2$ or more, or a BMI of 35 to 40 with comorbidities. Weight loss ranged from 50 kg to 100 kg over 6 to 12 months.

There is a much lower risk of rebound weight gain compared with other modes of weight-reduction treatment, because of the permanent nature of the intervention. The risks of mortality and morbidity accompanying obesity increase with the degree of overweight, so the management of severe or morbid obesity assumes greater importance, and for such patients the surgical option is an important alternative.

The advent of laparoscopic techniques has considerably reduced the operative risk and the financial costs, allowing such surgery to become more widely available.

> **Box 8.1**
>
> Current thinking is that 'the benefits (of gastrointestinal surgery for severe obesity) outweigh the risks and that this more aggressive approach is reasonable in individuals who strongly desire substantial weight loss and have life-threatening comorbid conditions'.[2]

Surgery for obesity is becoming more popular in the USA. The 40 000 operations performed in the year 2000 amounted to twice the number carried out in 1995.[3] In contrast, few such operations have been performed in the UK – current estimates are less than 200 per year, and many of these are funded privately.[4] In the UK, the number of obesity surgeons fell from 38 in 1991 to 23 in 1998.[5] An unpublished survey found that there were 12 obesity clinics in England in 1998, eight of which were run by physicians and four by surgeons.[6]

Aims of surgery

The goal of obesity surgery is to induce and maintain the loss of at least half of the excess body weight, to improve health-related quality of life, and to reduce obesity-related morbidity and mortality.

The National Institute for Health in the USA recognises surgery as being an effective treatment for morbidly obese patients.[3]

Patient selection

Patient selection is primarily a matter of clinical judgement by the practitioners involved. However, it is widely recommended that weight-loss surgery should be restricted to patients who desire substantial weight loss due to their poor quality of life, and who have a BMI of 40 kg/m^2 or more, or a BMI of 35 kg/m^2 or more if the patient has dangerous comorbidities such as severe heart disease. In exceptional cases, individuals with a BMI of 35 kg/m^2 may be considered as candidates for surgery in the absence of comorbidities if they have an extremely poor family history of early mortality from ischaemic heart disease or early-onset diabetes.[1]

It is estimated that 50% of the morbidly obese population could be suitable for surgery.[7]

Patients usually receive multidisciplinary screening prior to undergoing surgery. Each individual is given a thorough medical and psychological assessment to ascertain his or her suitability for the procedure. Most patients will already have been investigated in primary care or hospital obesity clinics, but will have further biochemical and metabolic screening performed, as well as sleep studies if appropriate, and standard pre-operative tests. They will be offered further dietary and lifestyle advice, and also behavioural therapy, and will be expected to lose 10% of their body weight measured from the moment they first sought medical advice prior to surgery being considered.

Psychological and psychiatric assessment is an integral part of the pre-operative screening process for the following reasons.

1 There is an increase in the prevalence of psychiatric and psychological conditions in grossly obese patients, including depression, low self-esteem and suicidal ideation. It is essential to diagnose and treat such conditions before embarking on surgery, and to refer such patients for alternative therapy as appropriate. Post-operative problems may result if pre-existing depressive disorders do not resolve as expected, so it is better to address such problems beforehand.

2 The psychological implications of weight-loss surgery for an individual are immense. It is important that patients are well informed and counselled about what they are letting themselves in for. Then it is necessary to assess whether or not they have the temperament and psychological stability to deal with the operation and its aftereffects. Some patients are so desperate to lose weight at any cost that they may not have given much thought to their 'life after surgery' when they are physically unable to eat a meal above a certain size, or to eat certain foods without discomfort.

It is a major step for an individual to surrender control of their weight to another person. Whilst being managed by conservative methods, a patient can still choose whether to comply with the treatment or to stop dieting for a day or even altogether, to catch the bus to work instead of walking, or to miss a pill. The last voluntary act a patient undertakes is to sign the consent form for surgery and submit to the anaesthetic. Thereafter the surgeon has control, and there is a permanent change in the patient's bodily structure and function. For some patients this handing over of responsibility amounts to an admission of failure, while for others having someone else assume control represents a giant step forward in their treatment, and they are tremendously optimistic. Some individuals view their decision as a chance to deflect the blame on to someone else if they still do not lose weight.

Box 8.2 Selection criteria for surgery (adapted from International Federation for the Surgery of Obesity[5])

- BMI > 40 or $35-40 \, \text{kg/m}^2$ in patients with serious comorbidities that are treatable by weight loss.
- Being obese for a minimum of 5 years.
- Age between 18 and 55 years*.
- Acceptable operative risk.
- Unlikely future weight loss from conservative treatment.

* Age is not universally agreed to be a criterion for patient selection.

Those in primary and secondary care teams should anticipate the effects of surgery, try to prepare the patient beforehand, and provide both physical and psychological care and support in the aftermath of surgery. The patient will experience changes in body image and self-esteem and also changes in how they are viewed by their spouse, friends, relatives and the public. They may have problems coming to terms with the loss of personal freedom to eat and drink anything they want, to go out and enjoy a meal without restriction, and the possible unwanted side-effects of discomfort and vomiting.[7]

Patients who are unsuitable for surgery

Some patients may decide not to opt for weight-loss surgery following the screening and counselling processes, while others may be deemed unsuitable. The screening process may detect biochemical evidence of an undiagnosed cause of obesity, or individuals for whom non-invasive management is clearly a better option. Patients may lose sufficient weight as a 'pre-operative' measure, so that the operation is no longer necessary. In other individuals there may be a psychological or underlying psychiatric disorder which either needs alternative treatment, or at least needs to be dealt with before surgery is considered. Schizophrenia, personality disorder and uncontrolled depression are absolute contraindications to surgery. Individuals whose obesity is caused by love of food, or patients with conditions such as 'binge-eating' disorder, may find the adjustment of their behaviour post-operatively particularly difficult.

Prior to embarking on surgery, the risk–benefit ratio is considered, and the patient may be deemed unsuitable for surgery depending on their comorbidities, anaesthetic risk and general well-being. In addition to the usual operative risks, serious post-operative infection may occur. Surgery carries a mortality risk of up to 1%.[8]

Women of childbearing age are treated with extreme caution because the increased nutritional needs of pregnancy will be hampered by the reduced capacity for absorption of nutrients. Such patients are advised not to fall pregnant after surgery until their weight has stabilised and their micronutrient status has been checked.

Role of those working in primary care

The initial approach to the topic of weight-loss surgery should be made through primary care. GPs should be aware of the various operative techniques and their ramifications, especially the permanent nature of such procedures. They should know which patients are suitable for surgery and what the operative criteria are. Each potential candidate for surgery will have undergone first-line treatment by diet, lifestyle changes, behavioural therapy and usually drug therapy by the time they are ready to discuss surgery. The GP should be able to give the patient realistic expectations of weight-loss surgery – for instance, that they will probably lose about 50% of their excess weight but may still consider themselves to be overweight once their condition has stabilised.

Modes of surgical treatment[7]

Only experienced surgeons in special centres should perform these operations. The operation most widely used in Europe is gastroplasty, by gastroplication or gastric stapling. Gastroplasty is being increasingly performed laparoscopically.

Restrictive procedures

Gastroplasty

The term *gastroplasty* implies the changing of the shape of the stomach. This is done by partitioning a pouch of 15 to 40 mL at the top of the stomach, which rapidly fills with food, and then empties slowly through a narrow channel into the body of the stomach. The pouch restricts the volume of food that a person can eat by reducing the stomach's functional capacity.

The operation is referred to as *gastric stapling* because of the line of staples that is used to divide the stomach. The most commonly used procedure is the *vertical banded gastroplasty*, in which the pouch is formed along the line of the lesser curvature of the stomach and empties through a channel of about 11 mm diameter. The channel or stoma is externally wrapped or *banded* to prevent stretching or more rapid passage of food. Patients consume a liquid-only diet, supplemented by iron and vitamins, for around three months to avoid breakdown of the stapled joins. They then progress to a carefully balanced diet supervised by a dietitian and taken as small regular amounts throughout the day.

Laparoscopic gastric banding

This is a technique in which an adjustable band is wrapped round the outside of the stomach in order to prevent distension and restrict food intake. The degree of restriction is altered by increasing or decreasing the pressure through an epigastric or abdominal portal. The pressure alterations are made by the surgical team rather than the patient, who might increase the pressure by too much in order to facilitate more rapid weight loss, or by too little in order to be able to eat more.

These restrictive procedures are technically easy, have low morbidity, do not cause malabsorption (as food eventually passes through the gastrointestinal tract in the usual way), and cost less than other surgical procedures. However, the degree of sustained weight loss may not be as great as that achieved with other procedures. Some patients recognise that high-calorie liquids such as milkshakes, ice-cream and alcohol pass rapidly through the stoma without causing fullness, and they change their diet accordingly, thereby regaining weight. The alteration of pressure within the band can be an uncomfortable procedure, partly due to the increased restriction of the stomach, and partly because of the needle used to access the portal.

Gastric bypass or Roux-en-Y bypass

Gastric bypass surgery is widely used as a first-line procedure in obesity surgery. A 10 mL segment is isolated from the body of the stomach, but is surgically separated from the remainder of the organ and anastomosed to the proximal jejunum, bypassing most of the stomach and the entire duodenum. This restricts food intake in the same way as gastroplasty, as well as inducing a degree of malabsorption. This double action is what makes gastric bypass surgery so effective in inducing and maintaining long-term weight loss. Gastric bypass surgery is a larger and more technically demanding operation than gastroplasty, and malabsorption (especially of iron, folate and vitamin B_{12}) can occur post-operatively, requiring careful monitoring for life.

Jejuno-ileal bypass

This procedure was abandoned around 1980 because of the high rate of complications, although patients with late side-effects from the procedure may still be encountered in primary care. More than 90% of the small bowel was bypassed by attaching the beginning of the jejunum to the end of the ileum, leaving a total of only 18 functional inches. This caused rapid transit of food through the bowel, and incomplete digestion, leading to malabsorption and severe steatorrhoea. Subjects could eat an unrestricted diet with no change in eating habits and still lose weight. Those undergoing the operation did lose weight – often over half their excess weight – but complications were common and occasionally life-threatening. These complications included acute hepatic failure, cirrhosis, oxalate nephropathy and chronic renal failure, immune-complex arthritis and malabsorption syndromes. Surgical re-anastomosis may be required to limit the associated morbidity.

Surgery for 'super-obese' patients

Specialist forms of surgery have been designed for 'super-obese' individuals who have a BMI greater than $50 \, \text{kg/m}^2$, are at least 225% overweight or weigh more than 400 lb, with life-threatening obesity-related morbidity. These radical procedures involve 80% distal gastrectomy and gastro-ileostomy with diversion of biliary and pancreatic secretions to the distal ileum. This is said to result in intense weight loss with malabsorption, especially of the fat-soluble vitamins, folate, vitamin B_{12}, iron and calcium, all of which need to be monitored and if necessary supplemented.

Liposuction

This is is a cosmetic procedure that involves the suction of fatty material from under the skin by means of a trochar. Liposuction usually results in the removal of approximately 3 litres of fat, but has some-times involved the loss of up to 10–12 litres in extreme cases. Although the technique has occasionally been used as a treatment for morbid obesity, it does not normally result in the loss of sufficient fat to be considered in this category.

Jaw wiring procedures

These procedures are no longer recommended by some authorities. They have not been tested in a randomised controlled trial, but in one study of 17 obese patients, the significant amount of weight that was lost whilst the wires were in place was regained at an unusually rapid rate once the wires had been removed. The jaws are wired in such a way that the patient can drink but not chew. Strong fixation is needed to resist the strains on the wires caused by coughing or sneezing. Some practitioners have fitted waist cords once the jaw wiring has been removed, to limit the amount of weight regained. One study of 35 patients whose jaws were wired described the 14 patients who stayed the course and had waist cords fitted after the wires were removed as achieving an average weight loss of 33 kg over a period of three years.[7]

Apronectomy

This is not a treatment for obesity, but it is helpful for patients who have lost large quantities of weight and have overhanging folds of excess skin as a result. Other common sites for skin-contouring operations following weight reduction are the under-arm area (known as a *brachioplasty*), and the inner and outer aspects of the thighs. Abdominal apronectomy can be circumferential, involving skin removal round the patient's back. Male subjects may undergo gynae-comastia correction.

It can be psychologically damaging to deny patients such surgery on financial or other grounds after they have followed medical advice diligently, but are left feeling uglier with their hanging skin folds, and with lower self-esteem than when they started. Skin contouring is a technically straightforward procedure, and its satisfying results can help to maintain long-term weight loss.

Artificial bezoar

This procedure involves the insertion of a balloon or object into the stomach in order to decrease its capacity. It has not proved successful as a treatment for obesity.

Results of surgery

Patients can expect to lose an average of 50–60% of their excess body weight and a decrease in BMI of about $10 \, kg/m^2$ during the first one to two years after surgery, That is, they usually lose about 30–70 kgs over a period of 12–18 months after their operation.[8] This is often followed by a modest weight gain of 5–7 kg in subsequent years.

Weight loss is greater and better maintained following bypass surgery than after gastroplasty. Type 2 diabetes resolves in around 90% of patients, and hypertension resolves in two-thirds of cases. Serum HDL levels are improved and cholesterol and triglyceride levels are lowered. Other comorbidities improve in proportion to weight loss.

Box 8.3

One review of the outcomes of surgery in 14 000 patients on the International Register of Obesity Surgery, reported that the average weight loss was 53% of excess weight for vertical banded gastroplasty and 72% of excess weight for gastric bypass operations one year after surgery. The operative mortality was 1.2%.[9]

Dramatic improvements in health-related quality-of-life measures have been demonstrated following surgery, especially when obesity is related to psychological problems. The extent of improvements is directly proportional to the amount of weight lost.

Follow-up of patients who have undergone surgery for obesity has shown improvements in the following:

- quality of life
- cure for some patients with type 2 diabetes
- control of hypertension
- reduction in atheroma

- likelihood of employment
- healthcare costs (lower)
- lipid profiles
- sleep apnoea
- musculoskeletal problems
- oesophageal reflux
- urinary incontinence
- asthma.[7]

Reflection exercises

Exercise 16

Have you any patients who have undergone bariatric surgery under your care now or in the past? If so, undertake an audit to find out whether they are being followed up regularly (e.g. checking of their weight and full blood count to review their nutritional status at least annually).

Exercise 17

Do you know where to refer patients for surgical weight-loss therapy? Do you need to undertake further reading about the surgical management of patients who are morbidly obese? Do you feel competent to advise an obese patient whose BMI is greater than $40 \, \text{kg/m}^2$ about the risks and benefits of undergoing gastric surgery for their obesity? If not, re-read and reflect on this chapter and look up the references cited here for a more detailed consideration of the pros and cons of surgery and the risks of continuing obesity.

Draw up your action plan accordingly – including service development and learning activities.

Exercise 18

Can you imagine how desperate someone must feel to be prepared to undergo bariatric surgery with the subsequent discomfort and dietary limitations? Take some time to talk to several of your obese patients at future consultations (e.g. three people with BMI values greater than $40 \, \text{kg/m}^2$), and try to understand their individual situations and how they are regarded by others. Listen to their stories and what approaches they have tried, so that you can reach a negotiated agreement with them about future therapy by concordance (*see* page 79) rather than by compliance.

Now that you have completed these interactive reflection exercises, transfer the information to the empty template of the personal development plan on pages 141–151 if you are working on your own learning plan, or to the practice personal and professional development plan on pages 165–172 if you are working on a practice team learning plan. Don't forget to keep the evidence of your learning in your personal portfolio.

References

1 Balsiger B, Murr M, Poggio JL *et al.* (2000) Bariatric surgery. Surgery for weight control in patients with morbid obesity. *Med Clin North Am.* **84**: 477–89.

2 Garrow J and Summerbell C (2002) Obesity. In: *Health Care Needs Assessment.* Third Series. Radcliffe Medical Press, Oxford.

3 Charatan F (2001) Obesity surgery grows in popularity in the US. *BMJ.* **321**: 980.

4 Department of Health (2001) *Consultation Letter in Relation to Appraisal of Surgery as Therapy for the Grossly Obese by the National Institute for Clinical Excellence.* Department of Health, Leeds.

5 Baker M (2001) *Official Response from the Royal College of General Practitioners to the National Institute of Clinical Excellence in Respect of Surgery for Obesity.* Royal College of General Practitioners, London.

6 National Audit Office (2001) *Tackling Obesity in England.* National Audit Office, London.

7 Garrow J (1999) Surgical treatments. In: *Obesity. Report of the British Nutrition Foundation Task Force.* Blackwell Science, Oxford.

8 Lean M (1998) *Clinical Handbook of Weight Management.* Martin Dunitz, London.

9 Mason E, Tang S, Renquiat K *et al.* (1997) Decade of change in obesity surgery. *Obesity Surgery.* **7**: 189–97.

CHAPTER 9

Calculating the costs of overweight and obesity

Ian Campbell

As the prevalence of obesity is rising so rapidly, the cost to our national resources is immense. In the UK the economic cost of overweight and obesity and the associated comorbidities represents more than 4% of National Health Service expenditure.[1]

This is lower than in some other countries. The direct costs of diagnosis and treatment of overweight and obesity and its comorbidities have been estimated to be up to 8% of total healthcare expenditure in the USA and other developed countries.[2,3] A study conducted in Australia in 1990 estimated their direct costs to be A$395 million. In the same year in France direct costs were estimated to be FF12 billion, and reports from Sweden, The Netherlands, Finland and elsewhere in Europe have described similar findings.[4] It is difficult to make international comparisons, as differing definitions of clinical obesity influence the prevalence and incidence figures for particular countries, and cost-of-illness studies are based on prevalence and incidence.

Cost-of-illness studies of obesity estimate the financial and social burden on society as a whole and on the individual. Indirect or societal costs relate to the consequences of overweight and obesity, such as absenteeism from work and lost productivity. There are social costs, too, which are measured in terms of human suffering. Thus the costs of failing to treat overweight and obesity cannot be judged only in financial terms.

Costs of obesity management in the NHS

The strategies that are being developed for obesity management services in the NHS at practice and district levels will undoubtedly impact on practice resources and practitioners' workloads. The introduction of new pharmacological treatments such as orlistat and sibutramine, and their likely usage rates, must be anticipated when planning and costing the best management options for patients.

The evaluation of such treatments and the strategic decisions that are made about the management of obesity should take into account not only the clinical efficacy of the various treatment options, but also the estimated costs of *not* treating obesity. The extent and types of comorbidities that are experienced by people who are overweight or obese have been discussed in previous chapters, and they cannot be neglected in any estimation of the costs of non-treatment.

When attempting to cost the treatment of obesity, consider the direct costs, the indirect costs and the intangible costs. Direct costs accounted for nearly one-fifth of all costs when direct and indirect costs of treating obesity were totalled for England in 1998. The total was £2.6 billion, or 0.3% of the gross national product.[3]

Direct costs

These include the costs incurred by a healthcare system in diagnosing and treating obesity, such as expenditure on staff salaries, support infrastructure, primary care and hospital services, drugs and medical supplies, emergency services and rehabilitation services. Direct costs also include costs accrued by patients themselves – for alternative travel, added help at home, dietary products, commercial weight loss programme attendance and clothing.[5]

A conservative estimate of the direct healthcare costs of obesity and overweight in the NHS in England in 1998 was around £500 million,[3] equivalent to about 1.5% of NHS expenditure in that year. This excluded such costs as treating obesity-related depression and hyperlipidaemia. Table 9.1 shows that the costs of treating the consequences of obesity – the secondary diseases attributable to the obesity – accounted for about 98% of the total costs.

Increased prescribing of the newly available anti-obesity drugs will initially only increase these direct costs. Based on the manufacturer's estimate, the total annual drug costs incurred by implementing the NICE guidelines for prescribing the anti-obesity drug orlistat in England

Table 9.1 Estimated direct costs of treating obesity and its consequences in England in 1998

Cost component	Estimated cost (£ million)
Treating obesity	
GP consultations	6.8
Ordinary admissions	1.3
Prescriptions	0.8
Outpatient attendances	0.5
Day cases	0.1
Total direct costs of treating obesity	9.5
Treating the consequences of obesity	
Prescriptions	247.2
Ordinary admissions	120.7
Outpatient attendances	51.9
GP consultations	44.9
Day cases	5.2
Total direct costs of treating consequences	469.9
Total direct costs	479.4

and Wales will be in the region of £12 million in the first year. The costs of administering the drug will include more visits to GPs, dietitians and/or specialist clinics – and will probably amount to another £3–4 million per year, giving a total of £16 million. Although it is anticipated that there may be some savings as a result of effective weight management and additional prescribing of orlistat, it is difficult to quantify them. There is still uncertainty about the maintenance of weight loss in the longer term, and in particular about how long the weight loss may be sustained after discontinuing orlistat therapy.[5]

Box 9.1

To put this in context, the total cost of the private slimming industry in the UK is thought to be of the order of £1–2 billion per annum.[1]

As regain of weight after healthcare interventions is common, the investment in consultations, investigation and treatments for managing obesity is mainly wasted in terms of sustained gains in quality of life and reduced disability.

Any successful population-based programme that aims to reduce the incidence and prevalence of obesity and overweight in future will involve national costs such as investing in cycle paths or safe walking areas, more accessible leisure facilities, effective educational approaches for children and adults, recruitment and training of additional dietitians, etc.

Indirect costs

It is difficult to calculate indirect costs exactly. They include the costs to society of production losses due to illness, disability or premature death resulting from obesity, such as increased social benefit payments, earlier pensionable retirement age, and the loss of commercial and service industry production. Lower levels of educational achievement and poorer employment opportunities are also significant indirect costs.

Chronic non-fatal disease due to overweight and obesity accounts for much higher indirect costs than premature mortality, because of the far larger numbers of people involved and the long period of time for which they are affected.

The association between obesity and the likelihood of being too disabled to work becomes stronger the greater the degree of obesity. The rates of pensionable work disability in men increase from 9.2 per 1000 men with a BMI of 22.5 kg/m² (in the ideal range) to 12.4 per 1000 men with a BMI of 30 kg/m² (obese). Similarly, 6.3 per 1000 women with a BMI of 22.5 kg/m² have a work disability pension, compared with 12.2 per 1000 women with a BMI of 30 kg/m².[6]

The National Audit Office report gave a cautious estimate of the indirect costs of obesity as totalling £2.1 billion in England in 1998, and indicated that the real figure could be much higher.[3] Nearly two-thirds of this figure (£1.3 billion) was due to sickness absence attributable to obesity, and the rest (£0.8 billion) was due to premature mortality. Translated into actual figures, this represents 18 million sick days and 40 000 lost years of working life per annum.

In 1992, a Swedish study estimated that obesity accounted for a total productivity loss of 7%, and in the USA in 1986 indirect costs were put at US$20 billion. The figures will have risen significantly since then.[4]

Finland has well-documented information about the indirect costs of obesity. About a quarter of all disability pensions are due to cardio-vascular and musculoskeletal causes in women, and about one-sixth of disability pensions in men have been attributed to overweight (BMI greater than 25 kg/m^2) alone. It is likely that other developed countries, such as the UK, have similar patterns.[4]

Intangible costs

These costs are in essence incalculable, but they represent a significant amount of human suffering which cannot be quantified in financial terms. Examples include personal costs such as psychological distress, loss of self-esteem, physical pain, and loss of employment and travel opportunities that result from obesity. Social isolation (either by choice or as a result of social stigma) and relationship difficulties are other intangible costs.

Box 9.2

A UK study found that obese women earned on average 10% less than non-obese women.[2] Women who were obese at the age of 23 years earned 5.3% less than women who were not obese at that age. The earnings of obese and non-obese men did not differ. Other studies have demonstrated this significant inverse relationship between obesity and earnings for women.

Treating obesity

Obesity is both a significant burden on our National Health Service resources and a cause of much morbidity and suffering. We need to invest in better, more accessible weight-management programmes for our patients, and we need to make the right tools for obesity management available through training initiatives.

One report has estimated that effective interventions to reduce and sustain weight loss in those who are overweight or obese might reduce healthcare expenditure in England by up to £131 million per annum (at 1996 prices) for patients with a BMI threshold of 25, or £15 million for those with a BMI threshold of 30. The authors emphasise the import-ance of targeting effective interventions at people who are overweight, and not just those who are obese.[7]

Most of the expenditure on obesity in the UK is incurred by GPs, practice nurses or dietitians giving advice about diet as part of face-to-face consultations. For instance, one-third of dietitians' total contact time cost is spent on weight management, as opposed to diabetes or dyslipidaemia.[6,7] Research findings have suggested that there would be greater cost-benefits if the NHS targeted the same resources at fewer patients with more effective treatments.[7]

In order to develop a continuing analysis of the financial implications of obesity, its comorbidities and the cost of treatment, credible cost-of-illness studies are necessary to raise awareness of the problem among governments, healthcare workers and the public. Equally, convincing economic evaluations of the various treatment modalities that are available will help decision makers to determine the best courses of action to take to enable physicians to manage obesity with appropriate therapies.[4]

If the prevalence of obesity continues to rise at the present rate, the annual direct and indirect costs of obesity are expected to rise by over one-third by 2010, which would mean a total of £3.6 billion for England alone.[3]

Reflection exercise

Exercise 19

Think about the direct, indirect and intangible costs of the following two scenarios – consider the costs now and the likely costs in 20 years' time.

1   An obese middle-aged woman with a BMI of 34 kg/m² who sees the GPs in her practice at least monthly with a variety of apparently obesity-induced symptoms, namely backache, osteoarthritis of the knees, incontinence and depression. One GP weighed her once a year ago, but alluding to her weight at that time triggered tears, and he has avoided remarking on her obesity since then. She has recently asked to try drug therapy for her obesity.
2   A 30-year-old man with a BMI of 39 kg/m², whose mother has type 2 diabetes. He sees the GP or practice nurse about once a year if he has an acute infection, or for travel immunisations, etc. Apart from some brief opportunistic advice to quit smoking he has not been given any lifestyle advice.

How can you revise your practice weight-management protocol or the way in which you apply it in your practice so that you intervene more effectively at an earlier stage before expending costs on treating the consequences of obesity?

Now that you have completed this interactive reflection exercise, transfer the information to the empty template of the personal development plan on pages 141–151 if you are working on your own learning plan, or to the practice personal and professional development plan on pages 165–172 if you are working on a practice team learning plan. Don't forget to keep the evidence of your learning in your personal portfolio.

References

1 Lean M (1998) *Clinical Handbook of Weight Management*. Martin Dunitz, London.

2 McIntyre A (1998) Burden of illness review of obesity: are the true costs realised? *R Soc Health*. **118**: 76–84.

3 National Audit Office (2001) *Tackling Obesity in England*. National Audit Office, London.

4 Malek M (2000) Cost-of-illness studies in obesity. *Obesity Pract*. **2**: 2–5.

5 National Institute of Clinical Excellence (2001) *Guidance on the Use of Orlistat for the Treatment of Obesity in Adults*. National Institute of Clinical Excellence, London.

6 Garrow J (1999) Treatment of obesity. VII. Resources and evaluation. In: *Obesity. Report of the British Nutrition Foundation Task Force*. Blackwell Science, Oxford.

7 Garrow J and Summerbell C (2002) Obesity. In: *Health Care Needs Assessment*. Third Series. Radcliffe Medical Press, Oxford.

CHAPTER 10

Draw up and apply your personal development plan focusing on motivation and lifestyle change management

You may want to focus on the management of obesity in general, or you may be interested in a specific aspect, such as motivation or lifestyle change management. A personal development plan (PDP) on any of these topics could form part of a practice personal and professional development plan (PPDP) (*see* Chapter 11). We have included a worked example of a personal development plan focused on learning about motivation and lifestyle change management on pages 128–140.

As we explained in the introduction, you may decide to allocate 50% of the time you intend to spend drawing up and applying a personal development plan in any one year to learning more about the effective management of obesity, including assessing people's readiness to change, motivation and lifestyle change management. That would leave space in your learning plan for other important topics such as diabetes, mental healthcare or cancer – whatever is a priority for you, your practice team and your patient population. There will be some overlap between topics, as you cannot consider a person with obesity in isolation from their mental health and general well-being or other associated comorbidities.

The worked example focused on motivation and lifestyle change management that starts on page 128 is very comprehensive, and you may not want to include so much detail in your own personal development plan. You might have a different approach and other educational activities, because your needs and circumstances are different to those of the example practitioners here. You might move on to Chapter 11, and modify the worked example of a practice personal and professional development plan focused on learning more about the management of obesity for your personal development plan.

Choose several methods to justify the topic you have chosen, or to identify your learning needs. Incorporate learning needs or baseline information from the 'Reflection exercises' at the end of each chapter, such as the clinical governance checklist from the material in Chapter 2, or the SWOT analysis in Chapter 1. Transfer the information about your learning needs from any of the reflection exercises at the end of the chapters that are relevant to you and that you have completed to the empty template of the personal development plan that follows on pages 141–151. The reflection exercises that you decide to select will depend on your learning needs and the focus of your personal development plan, as in the worked example here.

Draft your action learning plan. You might already have partly prepared this in one of the reflection tasks at the end of the chapters. Show it to someone else and ask for their views as to whether it is relevant, well balanced and achievable. Undertake your learning and demonstrate the subsequent improvements in your knowledge and practice.

Drawing up your personal development plan and carrying it out might take 10 to 20 hours depending on what topic you choose, the extent of the preliminary needs assessment you carry out, how detailed your action learning plan is and the type of evaluation that you do.

Worked example

Personal development plan focusing on motivation and lifestyle change management

Who chose the topic?
You may have chosen the topic yourself, but others in the practice may also have suggested that you take a lead in motivating patients to change their adverse lifestyle habits.

Why is the topic a priority?

(i) *A personal or professional priority?* You may not be familiar with the most up-to-date and effective approaches to help patients to lose weight or stop smoking. You might want to invest time and effort in health promotion to prevent ill health.

(ii) *A practice priority*? You will want to implement the most cost-effective ways to encourage patients to lose weight or deliver smoking cessation – and you may need to find out more.

(iii) *A district and/or national priority*? Obesity is a risk factor for diabetes, hypertension and cardiovascular disease, all of which are probably priorities in your district's health improvement programme (HImP).

Who will be included in your personal development plan?

You might include the following:

- GP colleague
- practice nurse
- health visitor
- community pharmacist
- dietitian
- receptionist to represent non-clinical staff.

(Although your personal development plan is about what *you* will learn, liaise with all of these people to agree a practice protocol and disseminate what you learn.)

What baseline information might you collect and how? How will you identify your learning needs?

You could ask the practice manager to find out details of what training is available in motivating people to change adverse lifestyle habits.

Find out from the primary care organisation (PCO) or local health promotion department if there are plans for any 'motivating people to change' initiatives, such as reducing overweight or smoking cessation, in your area. They may have a 'model' for personal change management that you could incorporate into your practice protocols.

Undertake an audit to find out how many of the patients you have advised to reduce overweight in the past have (A) lost some weight and (B) sustained that loss. Set aside the notes of the next 30 patients who consult you, who are at risk of developing coronary heart disease or who have established heart disease (e.g. those with hypertension, diabetes, or a strong family history of heart disease). How many of them are currently overweight or obese? How many have been recorded as being overweight or obese in the past (e.g. more than one year ago)? How much weight have they lost or gained now compared with the last measurement? Did you record giving them any advice about weight management? Did your approach at that time match the current practice protocol?

A parallel case-notes audit might establish the number of over-weight or obese patients for whom you played a contributory part in helping them to reduce their weight. Ask both those that have and those that have not lost weight if they remember you giving them advice in the past – and whether they can remember what you said, if you motivated them to try to reduce their weight, or what literature you gave them.

Read up on how to motivate people to change adverse lifestyle habits. How much did you know already and how much do you have to learn? Can you learn enough from reading, or do you need personal tuition or a visit to a practice that has best practice in place?

Ask colleagues how well they think you perform in relation to changing patients' behaviour. They may have some insight into how good you are at motivating patients to change, having heard their feedback at subsequent consultations.

What are the learning needs of the practice and how do they match your needs?

The reflection exercises earlier in the book should already have given you some information about your learning needs and those of the rest of the practice team. You may be focusing on learning more about motivating people to change, but you will also need to consider whether you or others have the computer skills necessary to set up templates for recording patients' body mass indices and smoking status, and for running audits. If no one in the practice has these skills, you should include IT training in your personal development plan. If others do have these skills, ask them to teach you what you need to know, and delegate other tasks.

Consider undertaking a SWOT analysis of the practice team's strengths, weaknesses, opportunities and threats with regard to motivating patients to change adverse lifestyle habits at a team meeting. You will start to gauge the extent of the practice's learning and organisational needs, so that you develop a systematic approach to motivating people to change for all your practice population. This SWOT exercise will help to identify your personal learning needs in relation to those of the practice team, and will gain their ownership of the initiative, too. For instance, you could consider the following points in the SWOT analysis.

Strengths: enthusiasm; willingness to learn (clinical evidence changes rapidly); good communication skills and inter-professional relation-ships that enable inter-disciplinary working; organisational, teaching and research skills to provide a resource for motivating people to change, once learned.

Opportunities: a GP or practice nurse in a neighbouring practice may have been on an updating course about weight management and be enthusiastic to pass on his or her newly acquired knowledge. The local pharmacist might have been trained in smoking cessation and could share what he or she learned about how to motivate people to change.

Weaknesses and threats: deficiencies of follow-up care in your practice organisation; poor record keeping by one or two clinical team members; little availability of training locally; other commitments, antagonism or lack of support from others; other staff being away on courses or involved with administrative tasks, so fewer people are available for routine work – and they may not be supportive of the additional time it takes for you to motivate patients to change in normal consultations; lack of time for health promotion, as staff are swamped by patients with acute illnesses.

Is there any patient or public input to your personal development plan?

Do you have a patients' group that wants to be involved in helping to give you feedback on what you individually or you as a practice team need to learn, or how best to apply your learning about motivating people to change? Could you ask them if they want a practice website, for example, containing information about staying healthy or losing weight?

Hold a roadshow in the practice one evening or on a Saturday morning on the topic of reducing weight or stopping smoking, and advertise it widely. Interested patients who attend will probably give you ideas about how the practice and the staff could improve the services, systems and procedures from a patient's perspective.

Consider the mechanism(s) that you will use to find out patients' views in a meaningful way – and not just the views of the most opinionated or most compliant! You may need to think deeply about the reliability of any method, and how representative individual respondents are of your whole practice population.

What are the aims of your personal development plan arising from the preliminary data-gathering exercise?

To learn how to motivate patients who are obese or overweight to change their lifestyle and sustain weight loss, and to apply that learning in practice.

How might you integrate the 14 components of clinical governance into your personal development plan focusing on motivating overweight or obese patients to change their lifestyle and lose weight?

> As you work through this clinical governance check-list, identify what learning needs you have to match the service needs you identify, and shape your action learning plan accordingly. These needs might include learning more about time management, communication and negotiation to enable you to function more effectively within the team, as well as specifically focusing on motivation and change with regard to improving weight management.

Establishing a learning culture: hold regular meetings (e.g quarterly) on clinical topics that you have prioritised where there are modifiable risk factors. Share what you learn about motivating patients to change with other practice team members, so that you transfer your new skills and information.

Managing resources and services: review whether you are prioritising patients who are overweight or obese and who have osteoarthritis, established heart disease or diabetes for advice about and treatment of their weight problem, and also review how you manage inter-team referrals of patients who need specialised advice and support to lose weight.

Establishing a research and development culture: disseminate information about the evidence base for effective interventions throughout the practice team (including the attached staff), and challenge current practices.

Reliable and accurate data: enter data about body mass index once, consistently and correctly, be able to retrieve it for a variety of uses, and be able to compare the data with other figures. Lead your practice in deciding on and using consistent Read codes, or in transferring to SNOMED.

Evidence-based practice and policy: find out which interventions are most successful and the evidence for motivating patients to change – use *Bandolier* and the York Centre for Reviews and Dissemination for updates (*see* list of websites in Appendix 1).

Confidentiality: ensure that you and others use passwords on the computer correctly and securely, and develop a policy to cover the issues.

Health gain: there are immense health gains for people who are successful in sustaining weight loss. Specific particular groups such as those who are physically disabled will really benefit if the weight loss makes a substantial difference to their mobility and independence.

Coherent team: every team member should be clear about their roles in advising and referring patients who want to reduce overweight or obesity, and should give consistent messages about the most effective approaches (e.g. recommending realistic weight-loss targets).

Audit and evaluation: set up regularly repeating audits to follow up outcomes of attempts to modify risk factors. Do not forget to include those patients who are more difficult to reach, such as those who are resident in continuing-care homes. It is never too late to promote weight management and help patients to reap the benefits of weight loss.

Meaningful involvement of patients and the public: consider running a patient focus group to gather patients' views about the services provided by the practice. If you do not know how to run such a group and obtain meaningful information, incorporate that learning into your action plan, too.

Health promotion: target patients with foot problems who are over-weight or obese, to promote weight loss. Other 'at-risk' groups you might focus on include patients with diabetes or coronary heart disease. Target these patient groups opportunistically, with specific reminders on their records as the latter are summoned up on the computer screen during a consultation. If you do not know what constitutes 'at risk' or how to operate the computer in this way, include those elements in your learning plan.

Risk management: young people who are overweight or obese and who already have chronic backache would be a good group to select for weight management. Patients with a family history of diabetes are another 'at-risk' group – weight reduction has the potential to prevent their developing type 2 diabetes. You could start by targeting these groups in order to practise your newly learned skills in motivating people to change. Agree a protocol to this effect with the practice team.

Accountability and performance: include your personal development plan and a record of the subsequent improvements you make in your portfolio, ready for revalidation or accrediting professional development (e.g. the Royal College of General Practitioners' Accredited Professional Development for GPs). You should be able to demonstrate how effective your learning has been. Review a sample of those patients whom you advise or treat for their overweight or obesity 12 months later. How many of them have sustained their weight loss?

Core requirements: could you work out a better skill mix in your practice team to provide a more cost-effective use of staff time that is spent on motivating patients to change adverse lifestyle habits such as poor diet and lack of exercise?

Action learning plan

Timetabled action. Start date: . . .

By 2 months: preliminary data gathered and colleagues working with you identified. The following information has also been obtained:
- Skills that are already present (your own, in practice, in the primary care organisation (PCO), health promotion department in health authority, etc.).
- Equipment and systems that are available (your own, in practice, in the PCO, outside in a training venue).
- Training that can be obtained to match your needs (in practice, at other practice(s), by distance learning, at some other local or distant venue), and how (private study, individual or group; tutor led or cascade learning).

By 4 months: review current performance.
- Review the results of audits of how well you are able to motivate patients to change their behaviour and reduce weight and/or sustain weight loss.
- Review what proportion of your practice population has had their BMI recorded. You might want to target high-risk groups first (e.g. those with diabetes or heart disease).
- Look at the opportunities arising from your SWOT analysis, and consider the weaknesses that you need to learn to rectify.
- Does the practice computer meet the specifications both for the tasks you are required to perform now and for those that you anticipate performing in the immediate future?

By 6 months: identify solutions and associated learning needs.
- Arrange the necessary training.
- Make a business plan for any associated equipment needs (e.g. a

computer program that calculates modifiable personal risks and benefits of change/weight loss).

- Arrange cover for yourself and any other staff who are involved, to provide protected time for learning.

By 12 months: make the changes and put your learning into practice.
- Implement the new systems or procedures.
- Obtain feedback from patients and other staff with regard to their impact.
- Iron out any difficulties.
- Identify any gaps in your knowledge and skills or the support services for motivating patients to change their diet and exercise habits.

Expected outcomes: more patients (set the exact target depending on your current baseline) with established heart disease or diabetes, and those at risk of heart disease, have their body mass index recorded; those who receive advice and help at the right time in the cycle of change are positively influenced (i.e. lose weight); motivating patients to change their lifestyle is incorporated into the practice protocol on weight management; practice team members understand their roles and responsibilities, with training needs fed into a practice-based learning plan; you apply best practice in motivating patients to change their behaviour; reliable, accurate data are easily entered, retrieved and then shared across the team.

How does your personal development plan tie in with your other strategic plans?

Diabetes and coronary heart disease are priorities for the PCO and the health improvement programme, so there should be local training programmes and resources to expedite learning and more effective motivation of patients to change their adverse lifestyle habits.

What additional resources will you require to execute your plan and from where do you hope to obtain them?

The PCO should be able to advise on how to access local resources (see above).

How will you evaluate your personal development plan?

Set specific objectives before starting, and compare at timed intervals what progress you are making. Set some learning objectives and some targets of actual benefits for patients (e.g. the number of patients who sustain agreed weight loss targets at 6, 12 and 24 months).

Also evaluate whether the type of learning activities you decided to pursue were the most appropriate ones in terms of what you aimed to learn (e.g. small group teaching might be better than a lecture for learning a behavioural modification skill).

How will you disseminate the learning from your plan to the rest of the practice team and patients? How will you sustain your new-found knowledge or skills?

Agree and monitor adherence to the practice protocol for weight management (e.g. at regular educational meetings where the topic is a relevant health problem, such as coronary heart disease).

How will you handle new learning requirements as they crop up?

Record them in your portfolio, as practice meeting notes, etc.

Check whether the topic you have chosen to learn is a priority and the way in which you plan to learn about it is appropriate.

> **Your topic:** *motivating patients to change their adverse lifestyles*

How have you identified your learning need(s) ?

(a) PCO requirement ☒   (e) Appraisal need ☐

(b) Practice business plan ☒   (f) New to post ☐

(c) Legal mandatory ☐   (g) Individual decision ☒
   requirement
    (h) Patient feedback ☐

(d) Job requirement ☐   (i) Other ☐

Have you discussed or planned your learning needs with anyone else?

Yes ☒   No ☐   If so, who? *Practice team.*

What are your learning need(s) and/or objective(s) in terms of the following?

Knowledge. What new information do you hope to gain to help you to do this?

Most effective interventions for motivating people to change lifestyle habits for weight management.

Skills. What should you be able to do differently as a result of undertaking this learning in your development plan?

Be able to offer effective advice to the right people at the right time and be able to motivate them to change their diet and exercise habits as appropriate.

Behaviour/professional practice. How will this impact on the way in which you subsequently do things?

I should be a more effective clinician, and be a more effective tutor to other staff about best practice with regard to weight management, smoking cessation, etc.

Details and date of desired development activity:

Add details of courses, etc., here.

Details of any previous training and/or experience that you have in this area/dates:

I attended a course on motivating people to stop smoking. That would involve learning and skills which I can transfer to helping overweight and obese people to lose weight.

What is your current performance in this area compared with the requirements of your job?

Need significant development in this area ☒   Need some development in this area ☐

Satisfactory in this area ☐   Do well in this area ☐

What is the level of job relevance that this area has to your role and responsibilities?

Has no relevance to job ☐   Has some relevance ☐

Relevant to job ☐   Very relevant ☒

Essential to job ☐

Describe how the proposed education/training is relevant to your job:

I should know how to motivate people to adopt healthier behaviour, and be able to demonstrate this skill by motivating and helping patients who are overweight or obese to lose weight and sustain that weight loss.

Do you need additional support in identifying a suitable development activity?

Yes ☒   No ☐

What do you need?

Practice manager is finding out about training opportunities.

Describe the differences or improvements for you, your practice, the PCO and/or NHS trust as a result of undertaking this activity:

It will be more likely that I recognise the stage at which overweight or obese patients are at present, and that I can therefore intervene more effectively.

Assess the priority of your proposed educational/training activity:

Urgent ☐   High ☒   Medium ☐   Low ☐

Describe how the proposed activity will meet your learning needs rather than any other type of course or training on the topic:

A one-day course will allow me to focus on the topic and learn practical skills.

If you had a free choice, would you want to learn this? Yes/No

If **No**, why not? (please circle all that apply)

Waste of time
I have already done it
It is not relevant to my work or career goals
Other

If **Yes**, what reasons are most important to you? (put them in rank order)

To improve my performance	2
To increase my knowledge	1
To get promotion	
I am just interested in it	
To be better than my colleagues	
To do a more interesting job	3
To enable me to be more confident	4
Because it will help me	
Other	

Record of your learning about motivating patients to change their adverse lifestyle

You would add the date, length of time spent, etc., for each learning activity

	Activity 1 – learning how to motivate people	Activity 2 – update IT skills	Activity 3 – revising the practice protocol
In-house formal learning	Share new understanding of motivating people to change, learned at external course (see below), at regular practice team learning event	Spend an hour with computer operator in practice to update skills on recording body mass index, writing that into practice protocol, and learning about running audits on computer	Rewrite protocol (with colleagues) for identifying and treating patients who are overweight or obese; organise inclusion of motivating patients to change in protocol
External courses	One-day course on motivating people to adopt healthier lifestyles		
Informal and personal	Reading and reflecting – articles in several months' issues of periodicals; look for relevant papers in professional journals; several informal chats with other staff about how they do this	Practise new-found computer skills using appropriate workbook (e.g. Gillies A (2000) *Information and IT for Primary Care.* Radcliffe Medical Press, Oxford)	Obtain feedback informally from users of the protocol about how it is working
Qualifications and/or experience gained	Certificate of attendance at course		Keep the protocol in portfolio, together with information about how it was produced

Reflection and planning exercise

Now complete your own personal development plan. It might be focused on a different topic to *motivating patients to change their adverse lifestyle.* It might be your personal perspective of the worked example of the practice personal and professional development plan focused on *weight management,* described in the next chapter.

Photocopy the template of a personal development plan that is given on the following pages, or complete the version in the book. Make a plan that meets your individual needs.

Template for your personal development plan

What topic have you chosen?

Who chose it?

Justify why this topic is a priority:

(i)   *A personal and professional priority?*

(ii)   *A practice priority?*

(iii) *A district priority?*

(iv) *A national priority?*

Who will be included in your personal development plan?
(Anyone other than you? GP colleagues, employed staff, attached staff, others from outside the practice, patients?)

What baseline information will you collect and how? How will you identify your learning needs?
(How will you obtain this information and who will do it? Self-completion check-lists, discussion, appraisal, audit, patient feedback?)

What are the learning needs of the practice and how do they match your needs?

Is there any patient or public input to your personal development plan?

What are the aims of your personal development plan arising from the preliminary data-gathering exercise?

How might you integrate the 14 components of clinical govern-ance into your personal development plan focusing on the topic of . . . . ?

As you work through this clinical governance check-list, identify what learning needs you have to match the service needs you identify, and shape your action learning plan accordingly. These needs might include learning more about time management, communication and negotiation to enable you to function more effectively within the team.

Establishing a learning culture:

Managing resources and services:

Establishing a research and development culture:

Reliable and accurate data:

Evidence-based practice and policy:

Confidentiality:

Health gain:

Coherent team:

Audit and evaluation:

Meaningful involvement of patients and the public:

Health promotion:

Risk management:

Accountability and performance:

Core requirements:

Action learning plan (include timetabled action and expected outcomes)

How does your personal development plan tie in with your other strategic plans?
(For example, the practice's business or development plan, the primary care investment plan or the health improvement programme)

What additional resources will you require to execute your plan and from where do you hope to obtain them?
(Will you have to pay any course fees? Will you be able to organise any protected time for learning in working hours?)

How will you evaluate your personal development plan?

How will you know when you have achieved your objectives?
(How will you measure success?)

How will you disseminate the learning from your plan to the rest of the practice team and patients? How will you sustain your new-found knowledge or skills?

How will you handle new learning requirements as they crop up?

Check whether the topic you have chosen is a priority and the way in which you plan to learn about it is appropriate.

Photocopy this proforma for future use.

Your topic:

How have you identified your learning need(s)?

(a) PCO requirement	☐	(e) Appraisal need	☐
(b) Practice business plan	☐	(f) New to post	☐
(c) Legal mandatory requirement	☐	(g) Individual decision	☐
		(h) Patient feedback	☐
(d) Job requirement	☐	(i) Other	☐

Have you discussed or planned your learning needs with anyone else?

Yes ☐   No ☐   If yes, who?

What are your learning need(s) and/or objective(s) in terms of the following?

Knowledge. What new information do you hope to gain to help you to do this?

Skills. What should you be able to do differently as a result of undertaking this learning in your development plan?

Behaviour/professional practice. How will this impact on the way in which you subsequently do things?

Details and date of desired development activity:

Details of any previous training and/or experience that you have in this area/dates:

What is your current performance in this area compared with the requirements of your job?

Need significant development in this area	☐	Need some development in this area	☐
Satisfactory in this area	☐	Do well in this area	☐

What is the level of job relevance that this area has to your role and responsibilities?

Has no relevance to job	☐	Has some relevance	☐
Relevant to job	☐	Very relevant	☐
Essential to job	☐		

Describe how the proposed education/training is relevant to your job:

Do you need additional support in identifying a suitable development activity?

Yes ☐   No ☐

If Yes, what do you need?

Describe the differences or improvements for you, your practice, your PCO and/or NHS trust as a result of undertaking this activity:

Assess the priority of your proposed educational/training activity:

Urgent ☐   High ☐   Medium ☐   Low ☐

Describe how the proposed activity will meet your learning needs rather than any other type of course or training on the topic:

If you had a free choice, would you want to learn this? Yes/No

If **No**, why not? (please circle all that apply)

Waste of time
I have already done it
It is not relevant to my work or career goals
Other

If **Yes**, what reasons are most important to you? (put them in rank order)

To improve my performance
To increase my knowledge
To get promotion
I am just interested in it
To be better than my colleagues
To do a more interesting job
To enable me to be more confident
Because it will help me
Other

Record of your learning activities

Write in the activity, date, time spent and type of learning

	Activity 1	Activity 2	Activity 3	Activity 4
In-house formal learning				
External courses				
Informal and personal				
Qualifications and/or experience gained				

Draw up and apply your practice personal and professional development plan focusing on obesity

The practice personal and professional development plan (PPDP) should cater for everyone who works in the practice. It will probably include health professionals who are attached to a practice, too. Clinical governance principles will balance the development needs of the population, the practice, the PCO *and* the individual personal development plans (PDPs) of your practice team.

You might want to start by asking everyone to identify their own learning needs, combining them with those of other people and then checking them against the practice business plan. Alternatively, you could start from the other direction, by developing a practice-based personal and professional development plan from your business plan and then identifying everyone's individual learning needs within that. Whichever direction you start from, you must ensure that you integrate team members' individual needs with those of your practice and the needs and directives of the NHS.

Make your learning plan flexible – you may want to add something in later when circumstances suddenly change or an additional need becomes apparent, perhaps as a result of a complaint, the launch of a new drug or new requirements from the Government, the PCO or the National Institute for Clinical Excellence (NICE).

Long-term locums (longer than six months, say), assistants, retained doctors and salaried GPs should all be included in the practice plan. Remember to include all those staff who work for the practice, however few their hours – you cannot manage without them or they would not be there!

Consider the time commitment when drawing up your action plan – be realistic and do not over-extend yourself. You should build in protected time during working hours so that education and training are not an 'add on' but an integral part of your working life.

Read through the worked example. It is not intended to be prescriptive, but merely a guide to the types of techniques that you might use to identify your learning needs, define your objectives, undertake an assessment against the 14 components of clinical governance, and plan your action and evaluation. Then turn to the empty template that follows and start to complete it by transferring the information you have gathered from the range of reflection exercises at the end of each chapter in the book.

Worked example

Practice personal and professional development plan focusing on management of overweight and obesity

Who chose the topic?

The practice team chose it, as they realised that they had not been targeting patients for weight management, and they wanted to develop a systematic approach instead of their current *ad-hoc* approach.

Justify why this topic is a priority?

(i) *A practice priority?* The practice team was being bombarded by patients requesting orlistat and other anti-obesity drugs. They wanted to review how to maximise the effectiveness of their prescribing policy. (ii) *A district and/or national priority?* The practice team was aware that weight management for those who are overweight or obese will help in their drive to improve the secondary prevention of cardiovascular disease, one of the targets for the National Service Framework for Coronary Heart Disease for England.

Who will be included in your practice personal and professional development plan?

The following might be included:

- GPs
- practice nurses
- practice manager

- receptionists
- district nurses
- community pharmacists
- health visitors
- local sports-centre staff
- community dietitian
- public and patients.

Who will collect the baseline information and how?

The practice manager might collect background information about current performance, others' perspectives, options for standards and guidelines that they might adopt, available resources, and sources of additional resources for the future.

Where possible, information could be requested from the primary care development manager of the PCO acting as a central resource for the information available within the PCO. The practice manager might organise receptionists and the practice secretary to help with the data collection.

The topic of weight management might link with parallel learning about coronary heart disease (CHD), hypertension, dyslipidaemias, and with reviewing standards of practice to determine gaps in services and associated learning needs.

You as a practice might collect information about the following:

- any previous or current practice-based initiatives to diagnose or treat overweight or obese patients – suggestions from patients/staff, minutes of practice meetings in the last 12 months which are relevant
- any recent audit of the proportion of patients who are particularly 'at risk' from their overweight or obesity because they also have diabetes or ischaemic heart disease or a family history of these conditions
- the objectives of the PCO's primary care investment plan
- practice-based prescribing data on anti-obesity drugs
- the health profile of the local community, local morbidity and mortality rates from the health authority – compare any practice-specific data with district figures
- any health needs survey that has already been undertaken by the local authority or health authority with regard to lifestyle habits
- published guidelines about weight management – compare your practice protocol with the guidelines from the National Obesity Forum (*see* Appendix 2) and decide whether you can justify any variations.

What information will you obtain about individual learning wishes and needs?

The practice manager might talk to representatives of the practice team individually about the demands of their posts, priorities, roles and responsibilities as part of appraisals. All members of the team could complete check-lists describing the following:

- their roles and responsibilities
- their own learning needs
- their comments on other team members' learning needs
- their ideas on how to improve advice giving and treatment for patients who are overweight or obese
- their personal aspirations and visions for the practice.

The practice manager could collate this material and discuss it with the practice leads on educational matters and clinical governance.

You might use any of the other methods for identifying and assessing learning needs as described throughout the reflection exercises in the book. For example, with regard to observing how other practices manage overweight and obesity, could one of the practice nurses or receptionists make an exchange visit with a member of staff in another practice to learn more about their systems?

What are the learning needs for the practice and how do they match the needs of the individual?

The effective management of overweight or obesity will include IT and audit skills, motivation and change management, and clinical management of overweight and obesity, as well as clinical effectiveness and evaluation. Individual staff members could propose themselves as candidates to learn more about any of these particular topics in areas where the practice is weak. For instance, the practice nurse could learn more about motivating patients to lose weight, or a secretary could learn more about efficient ways of managing practice disease registers.

Is there any patient or public input to your plan?

You might target patients who do not attend or who do not comply with the recommended treatment and find out why this is so by asking them directly.

You might set up a patient panel within your adult practice population by randomly selecting 30 patients from your practice list. Write to them and invite them to participate – either at occasional face-to-face meetings or via a quarterly postal survey. Ask them whether you have got the balance of your services right – whether they are convenient, accessible and appropriate. Ask questions that are relevant to patients who are overweight or obese.

How will you prioritise everyone's needs in a fair and open way?

A practice meeting might be devoted to the following:

- discussing and sorting all of the information about performance with regard to weight management
- the team members' views about possible improvements
- the importance of the learning needs that have been identified
- the priorities for the practice's development
- considering the impact of the PCO's plans
- the practice circumstances, aspirations and plans for changes to services.

A 'Hanging Committee' consisting of a GP, a nurse and the practice manager could then be convened to prioritise the educational plan for the practice to include the effective management of patients who are overweight or obese.

What are the aims of the practice personal and professional development plan arising from the preliminary data-gathering exercise?

To develop a learning programme that enables the practice team as a whole to adopt a systematic approach to helping patients who are overweight or obese to reduce their weight and sustain that weight loss, and to prioritise patients who have comorbidities or who are at risk of developing diabetes or ischaemic heart disease.

How might you integrate the 14 components of clinical governance into your practice personal and professional development plan focusing on the management of obesity and overweight?

As you work through this clinical governance check-list, identify what learning needs you have to match the service needs you have identified, and shape your action learning plan accordingly. These needs might include learning more about time management, motivation, communication and negotiation to enable you to function more effectively as a team, as well as improving your knowledge and skills of clinical management.

Establishing a learning culture: review the application of the practice protocol for managing overweight and obese patients – that is, address any gaps between theory (your protocol) and practice. This should involve all of the practice staff in multidisciplinary learning about their roles and responsibilities, from the receptionist who leads on the maintenance of the disease register to the GPs who update their everyday practice.

Managing resources and services: equipment should be regularly checked and in good order – check the consistency and reliability of the weighing scales in all of the consulting-rooms. Review the skill mix for any targeted initiatives for patients who are obese or overweight. Could a less qualified member of staff assume more responsibility or more of the workload?

Establishing a research and development culture: investigate whether there are any differences in the levels of treatment for obesity between men and women or between individuals in different ethnic groups in your practice.

Reliable and accurate data: establish a reliable way of identifying individuals who are overweight or obese and recording follow-up body mass indices so that you can offer patients the most effective treatment and monitor their response.

Evidence-based practice and policy: cite the evidence for prescribing anti-obesity drugs or referring for surgery to justify how you are spending your practice 'budget' according to recommended guidelines for best practice.

Confidentiality: patients should give their informed consent before being subjected to any activities outside usual NHS practice, such as taking part in any research study into the treatment or management of obesity, or being videotaped for educational purposes.

Health gain: there is a great deal of evidence about how morbidity and premature mortality can be reduced by those who are overweight or obese sustaining a weight loss of 10% or more. Osteoarthritis, hypertension, diabetes and other medical conditions can all be positively influenced by such weight reduction.

Coherent team: good teamwork is essential for managing patients who are overweight or obese, as their weight problem has an impact on all types of specialist care in the practice (e.g. the midwife with regard to antenatal care, the practice nurse with regard to diabetes care, the health visitor with regard to overweight children, the physiotherapist treating osteoarthritis and other joint problems, the community psychiatric nurse treating those whose weight problems accentuate their psychological problems, and the GP providing generalist care).

Audit and evaluation: undertake an audit to determine whether interventions are effective, rational and consistent, and whether patients adhere to treatment and advice.

Meaningful involvement of patients and the public: hold an open evening in the practice focusing on the theme of weight management, where you not only give patients as a whole more information about the problems that arise from being overweight or obese, but also invite patient feedback about your services. Act on this feedback so that it becomes 'meaningful', and make changes to your practice's systems and services as appropriate so that they are more accessible or delivered differently.

Health promotion: the promotion of exercise and a less sedentary way of life will reduce weight and decrease the risks of cardiovascular disease. Remind practice staff that this applies to them as well as to patients.

Risk management: prioritise patient groups for your efforts with regard to weight management, where their continuing overweight or obesity is increasing their risk of developing ischaemic heart disease or diabetes. Overweight children are another group to be prioritised where risk management is appropriate.

Accountability and performance: with the good teamwork that involves a wide range of staff from different disciplines all playing their part comes the need for clear lines of accountability.

Core requirements: organise education and training of practice staff to anticipate any change in the skill mix within the practice team and their need to know more about effective interventions in weight management.

Action learning plan

Who is involved?/What is the setting? Include the relevant people from the list on pages 154–155 – specify names, posts, timetabled action and start date.

By 3 months: preliminary data gathering and collation of baseline of providers.

- Is there a practice protocol for the management of overweight or obese patients? Is such management a component of other practice

protocols (e.g. for managing CHD, hypertension, screening for and control of cholesterol, diabetes, etc.)?
- Numbers of staff; map their expertise; list other providers.
- Referral patterns to dietitian, psychologist or surgeon because of obesity.
- Information about the characteristics of those recorded on the practice computer as being overweight or obese, including a breakdown by gender, age and coexisting conditions (e.g. diabetes, hypertension, osteoarthritis).
- Any relevant local and national priorities, and any additional associated resources for which you might apply.
- Staff report of problems that limit patients accessing services, problems observed, and views and suggestions from patients.

By 5 months: review current performance.
- Practice manager reviews links with services outside the practice that have an interest in or responsibility for obesity or overweight (e.g. private slimming clubs, sports centres, dietetics services).
- Clinical lead on obesity reviews the extent of knowledge and skills of the practice team with regard to routine care of patients who are overweight or obese.
- Audit actual performance against pre-agreed criteria (e.g. with respect to referrals, health promotion, management, investigation and patients' adherence to mutually agreed treatment plans).
- Compare performance with any or several of the 14 components of clinical governance (e.g. health promotion would be very relevant).

By 6 months: identify solutions and associated training needs.
- Set up new systems for access to services appropriate to people's needs.
- Give the practice team in-house training in effective interventions for overweight or obesity and the increased risks for patients with comorbidities.
- Revise the practice protocol after having undertaken a search for evidence, or after comparing others' evidence-based protocols with your own. Agree roles and responsibilities as a team for delivering care and services according to the protocol. Certain staff attend external courses, and the practice nurse or a GP provide some in-house training to other GPs and nurses.

By 12 months: make changes.
- Clinicians adhere to the practice protocol, as shown by repeat audits.
- Changed approaches to treatment are implemented, that are more appropriate for patients who are overweight or obese.

Expected outcomes: more effective prevention of obesity in general; improved adherence by patients to treatment and healthy lifestyle advice; revised practice protocol for weight management that is consistently incorporated into other practice protocols for hypertension and control of hyperlipidaemia and diabetes; ultimately lives are saved.

How does your practice personal and professional development plan tie in with your other strategic plans?

The practice team learning more about the effective management of overweight and obesity ties in with other priorities such as reduction of health risks in patients with coronary heart disease.

What additional resources will you require to execute your plan and from where do you hope to obtain them?

The practice might pay for the course fees of any member of staff who undertakes training that fulfils a priority need of the practice – as in this case with overweight and obesity.

You may be able to justify an application for additional resources to your PCO based on your preliminary learning and health needs assessments, tapping into the district or national strategic priorities.

If a member of staff is undertaking the training on behalf of the practice, the training should be undertaken in paid time if possible. Any learning that is cascaded to other members of the practice team as part of the practice personal and professional development plan should also be undertaken in paid time, and during working hours whenever possible.

How will you evaluate your practice personal and professional development plan?

The exact evaluation activities will depend on the aims and content of the learning plan. The practice might re-audit their management of overweight or obesity one year after setting out on the plan.

A SWOT analysis undertaken as part of the preliminary needs assessment will lend itself to review once the learning plan is in place or completed, in order to note the changes that have occurred and the extent to which 'weaknesses' have been redressed and 'threats' minimised.

Other evaluation techniques might include the observation of practice by someone who is independent of the team (e.g. from the local university), review of achievements during subsequent educational or job appraisals, or a repeat computer search to check developments with regard to recording of body mass indices.

How will you know when you have achieved your objectives?

Usually this will be by comparing the outcomes of your programme with baseline data. You should undertake your evaluation so as to be able to demonstrate the extent to which you have met the milestones you set out when devising your learning plan.

How will you disseminate the learning from your plan and sustain the developments and new-found knowledge or skills?

A member of the practice might attend the local community forum – where health matters and community safety are always on the agenda – to give and receive information relating to obesity among other health issues. One member of the practice team might write new literature for patients which also reminds others in the practice of the emphasis on the key messages and approaches to obesity that you have agreed.

A practice 'away-day' would provide a good opportunity to share learning and plan how to re-organise the practice team so as to provide more effective care of patients with obesity or associated comorbidities. Training could then be arranged for those who require additional knowledge and skills to fulfil their new roles and responsibilities with regard to the intended altered methods of working.

How will you handle new learning requirements as they crop up?

The practice manager might run audits at intervals and feed the results back to the practice team mid-way through the time period of the practice personal and professional development plan, when there is time to revise the activities.

Record of practice team learning about effective management of patients who are overweight or obese

You would add the date, length of time spent, etc., for each learning activity

	Activity 1 – establishing and maintaining a disease register for obesity	*Activity 2 – reviewing practice protocols*	*Activity 3 – employing appropriate and effective lifestyle interventions*	*Activity 4 – learning to work with local services in relation to obesity*
In-house formal learning	Practice development manager from the PCO spends 30 minutes of a practice meeting advising on new systems, after which the practice agree on who will do what, facilitated by the practice manager	Four weekly sessions reviewing protocols for overweight/obesity, hypertension, and controlling risks of coronary heart disease and diabetes, attended by GPs, nurses and practice managers; held with six local practices	Practice nurse and/or GP run small group session for others in the practice after attending the external course on how to motivate people to change	Set up a local half-day learning session, inviting representatives from private slimming clubs and the local sports centre, a dietitian, health visitors, community psychiatric nurse, community pharmacist and interested practice staff to discuss overlap and closer working
External courses			Practice nurse and GP attend day course on topic	Organise an open meeting for everyone in the practice population on overcoming overweight and obesity – with all those listed above contributing
Informal and personal	GPs and practice nurse read 'how to do it' in medical weekly newspaper, and then discuss how the suggested method would work in your practice, over tea/coffee. Later feed into in-house training (*see above*)	Discussion during in-house weekly sessions (*see above*) gives plenty of food for thought. Many participants at sessions do further reading in their own time to prepare for the next session	GP and nurse continue to reflect on how to apply what they have learned from the course to their practice setting	Discuss what the practice team learned over tea/coffee and how to utilise the available resources more consistently for priority groups of patients who would benefit most from weight reduction
Qualifications and/or experience gained	Record your learning – and subsequent changes in practice	Keep a record of your part in drawing up practice protocols	GP and nurse put course materials in their own portfolios	Record your learning and how you will use it

Reflection and planning exercise

Now build up and complete your practice personal and professional development plan. It might be focused on a number of topics in addition to tackling overweight and obesity. For instance, you might prioritise coronary heart disease or musculoskeletal disorders, too. Then you can mesh the personal development plans of everyone else in the practice team.

Photocopy the template of a practice personal and professional development plan that is given below, or complete the version in the book. Choose a topic that meets your individual practice needs.

The practice manager or a GP with responsibility for education might take a lead in this exercise. They will have to lead and motivate the team, anticipate skill needs for any planned changes in the way in which you will be approaching overweight and obesity management, and organise appropriate education and training in good time.

- Ensure that there are good communications within the practice about the learning plan.
- Organise regular staff meetings and separate educational meetings with team members and GPs. Invite attached staff to attend as appropriate.
- Be prepared to listen to staff and seek their involvement in changes.
- Agree protocols in clinical and organisational work practices and adhere to them.
- Monitor performance regularly and appraise staff. Move away from a blame culture, and use mistakes as learning opportunities (try anyway!).

Template for your practice personal and professional development plan

Photocopy the following pages and complete one chart per topic.

What topic have you chosen?

Who chose it?

Justify why this topic is a priority:
(i)   *A personal and professional priority?*

(ii) *A practice priority?*

(iii) *A district priority?*

(iv) *A national priority?*

Who will be included in the practice personal and professional development plan?
(GP colleagues, employed and attached staff, others from outside the practice, patients?)

What baseline information will you collect and how?

How will you identify your learning needs?
(How will you obtain this information and who will do it?
Self-completion check-lists, discussion, appraisal, audit, patient feedback?)

What are the learning needs of the practice and how do they match your needs?

Is there any patient or public input to your practice personal and professional development plan?

What are the aims of your practice personal and professional development plan arising from the preliminary data-gathering exercise?
(e.g. the reflection exercises throughout the book)

How might you integrate the 14 components of clinical governance into your practice personal and professional development plan focusing on the topic of . . . . ?

As you work through this clinical governance check-list, identify what learning needs practice team members have to match the service needs you identify, and shape your action learning plan accordingly. These might include learning more about time management, motivation, communication and negotiation to enable you to function more effectively as a team.

Establishing a learning culture:

Managing resources and services:

Establishing a research and development culture:

Reliable and accurate data:

Evidence-based practice and policy:

Confidentiality:

Health gain:

Coherent team:

Audit and evaluation:

Meaningful involvement of patients and the public:

Health promotion:

Risk management:

Accountability and performance:

Core requirements:

Action learning plan
(Include timetabled action and expected outcomes)

How does your practice personal and professional development plan tie in with your other strategic plans?
(e.g. the practice's business or development plan, the primary care investment plan or the health improvement programme)

What additional resources will you require to execute your plan and from where do you hope to obtain them?
(Will you have to pay any course fees? Will you be able to organise any protected time for learning in working hours?)

How will you evaluate your practice personal and professional development plan?

How will you know when you have achieved your objectives?
(How will you measure success?)

How will you disseminate the learning from your plan to the rest of the practice team and patients? How will you sustain your new-found knowledge or skills?

How will you handle new learning requirements as they crop up?

Record of your learning activities

Write in the topic, date, time spent and type of learning

	Activity 1	Activity 2	Activity 3	Activity 4
In-house formal learning				
External courses				
Informal and personal				
Qualifications and/or experience gained				

Sources of help

Organisations and websites

Bandolier. Website: www.jr2.ox.ac.uk/bandolier

British Dietetic Association, Fifth Floor, Elizabeth House, 22 Suffolk Street, Queensway, Birmingham B1 1LS. Tel: 0121 616 4900. Website: www.bda.uk.com

British Heart Foundation, 14 Fitzhardinge Street, London W1H 6DH. Tel: 020 7935 0185. Website: www.bhf.org.uk

The British Heart Foundation (BHF) and the Countryside Agency have begun a five-year 'Walking the Way to Health' initiative to encourage people who take little exercise to walk more in their own neighbourhoods. Further information is available. Tel: 01242 533258. Website: www.whi.org.uk

The BHF National Centre for Physical Activity and Health has recently produced a physical activity toolkit entitled *A Training Pack for Primary Health Care Teams*, which will shortly be distributed to all primary care groups in England, Scotland and Wales.

British Nutrition Foundation, High Holborn House, 52–54 High Holborn, London WC1V 6RQ. Tel: 020 7404 6504. Website: www.nutrition.org.uk

Community Practitioners and Health Visitors Association, 40 Bermondsey Street, London SE1 3UD. Tel: 020 7939 7000. Website: www.msfcphva.org

Diabetes UK, 10 Queen Anne Street, London W1G 9LH. Tel: 020 7323 1531. Website: www.diabetes.org.uk

Eating Disorders Association, First Floor, Wensum House, 103 Prince of Wales Road, Norwich NR1 1DW. Tel: 01603 621414. Website: www.edauk.com

Food Standards Agency, Room 621, Hannibal House, PO Box 30080, Elephant and Castle, London SE1 6YA. Tel: 0845 757 3012. Website: www.foodstandards.gov.uk

Health Development Agency, Trevelyan House, 30 Great Peter Street, London SW1P 2HW. Tel: 020 7222 5300. Website: www.hda-online.org.uk

Health Education Board for Scotland, The Priory, Canaan Lane, Edinburgh EH10 4SG. Includes the Health Promotion Library, Scotland. Tel: 0845 912 5442. Website: www.hebs.scot.nhs.uk

National Obesity Forum, PO Box 6625, Nottingham NG2 5PA. Tel/Fax: 0115 846 2109. Website: www.nationalobesityforum.org.uk

Overeaters Anonymous, PO Box 19, Stretford, Manchester M32 9EB. Tel: 07626 984674.

Overeaters Anonymous originated in America. It is a non-profit-making organisation which offers local group support for people who find it difficult to stop eating. There are 9000 groups in 52 countries. There is a national contact number. Tel: 07000 784985.

Royal College of Nursing, 20 Cavendish Square, London W1M 0DB. Tel: 020 7409 3333. Website: www.rcn.org.uk

Scottish Centre for Eating Disorders, 3 Sciennes Road, Edinburgh EH9 1LE. Tel: 0131 668 3051.

York Centre for Reviews and Dissemination. Website: www.york.ac.uk/inst/crd

National Obesity Forum guidelines for the management of adult obesity and overweight in primary care (reproduced with the permission of the National Obesity Forum)

There is a great deal of scientific and academic interest in the phenomenon of obesity. Unfortunately, this enthusiasm is not reflected in the standard of management of obesity and overweight in primary care. Instead, its importance is underestimated, and its treatment is neglected by the very people who can actually do something about it. Over 2000 pages of theoretical guidelines have been issued by the scientific community in the past few years. The National Obesity Forum has attempted to distil that information into two pages of guidelines, in order to form a useful basis for treatment during an ordinary consultation in primary care.

Patient selection

Active rather than passive; opportunistic screening rather than relying exclusively on self-referral; education of patients about the risks of obesity, using posters and leaflets in the surgery and community.

Box 1 Treatment groups

Treatment or advice should be offered to the following:

- patients with BMI $\geqslant 30 \, \text{kg/m}^2$
- patients with BMI $\geqslant 28 \, \text{kg/m}^2$ with comorbidities (e.g. chronic obstructed airways disease, ischaemic heart disease)
- patients with any degree of overweight coinciding with diabetes, other severe risk factors or serious disease
- patients who self-refer, where appropriate.

Investigations

The aims of these are as follows:

- to isolate any medical pathology
- to act as a baseline for future measurements
- to exclude any secondary conditions or comorbidities
- to reassure the patient that there is no reason why they cannot lose weight.

Height, weight, BMI ($\geqslant 25 \, \text{kg/m}^2$ overweight, $\geqslant 30 \, \text{kg/m}^2$, clinically obese), waist circumference ($> 102 \, \text{cm}$ for men, $> 88 \, \text{cm}$ for women associated with substantially increased health risk), blood pressure, urinalysis and blood tests if appropriate (thyroid function tests, liver function tests, blood sugar, cholesterol and triglycerides, hormone profile including cortisol, and sex hormones).

Other tests should be performed as dictated by comorbidities (e.g. chest X-ray, electrocardiogram, glucose tolerance test).

Primary care teamwork

After the initial assessment, management should involve as many members of the primary care team as possible, including the practice nurse, dietitian, etc., to provide supervision, motivation and advice about maintaining weight loss.

Treatment

Box 2 First-line treatment

- Motivation and encouragement (e.g. weight management clinics either within primary care or commercially run). Targets, treatments and expectations should be agreed with patients (e.g. 1–2 lb per week, or 10% of maintained weight loss rather than 'ideal weight'). Advice given about coexisting risk factors (e.g. alcohol, smoking, hyperlipidaemias). Regular follow-up appointments (e.g. 1 to 3 monthly for 1 year) to help to maintain weight loss.
- Permanent lifestyle changes: less television, computer games and sedentary lifestyles; more exercise, ideally 30–40 minutes of sustained exercise (e.g. brisk walking, swimming or cycling) at least 5 days per week.

Dietary changes

- *Quantitative*: reduce calorie intake by, for example, 500–600 kcal per day
- *Qualitative*: less dietary fat (e.g. 3 g fat per 100 g of food) and fewer 'empty calories' (e.g. avoid alcohol and chocolate); higher carbohydrate-to-fat ratio; regular meals; avoid eating just before bedtime.

The success of first-line treatment can be gauged after 3–6 months by the reduction in BMI, the percentage weight reduction (e.g. 10%), the improvement of symptoms, or by reduced markers of comorbidity (e.g. exercise tolerance or blood sugar levels). If these criteria are not achieved, then *second-line* treatment should be considered.

Box 3 Second-line treatment

- *Drug treatment*: the pancreatic lipase inhibitor orlistat may be used in conjunction with a low-fat diet to achieve more rapid and greater weight loss. Patients must lose 2.5 kg prior to treatment and demonstrate a 5% reduction in weight over three months in order to comply with licensing guidelines.

The centrally acting agent sibutramine may be taken for up to 12 months in conjunction with diet and exercise (*see* NOF website for latest guidance).
- *Behavioural therapy*
- *Alternative treatments*
- *Referral to secondary care, including various surgical procedures*: this can be extremely successful, but is only indicated in severely obese patients – that is, those who are $> 100\%$ above their ideal weight, have a BMI of $\geqslant 40\,kg/m^2$, or are at immediate risk of serious medical complications.

For further details, *see* http://www.nationalobesityforum.org.uk

Box 4

The National Obesity Forum (NOF) guidelines are drawn from other published guidelines (*see* Chapter 4) and the opinions of experienced primary care practitioners with regard to what constitutes a realistic approach at the 'coal-face' in general practice.

Index